UNDERSTANDING HIGH BLOOD PRESSURE

SIMPLE STEPS TO AVOID COMPLICATIONS, REDUCE
MEDICAL EXPENSES, DECREASE STRESS, AND LIVE A
HEALTHY & PROACTIVE LIFE

DR. ASHLEY SULLIVAN, PHARMD, RPH, MBA

CONTENTS

INTRODUCTION

> *"The doctor of the future will give no medication, but will interest his patients in the care of the human frame, diet and in the cause of prevention of disease"*

— THOMAS EDISON

If you or a family member have been diagnosed with high blood pressure, you have a family history, or are just interested in learning more—you're in the right place!

High blood pressure or hypertension is a disease that can gradually progress. It can put you at risk for a stroke, kidney disease, or a heart attack. So, what can you do to prevent these from happening? You'll find various lists of tips and advice online. However, it's not as easy as it seems with the mountain of information you need to go through, and not knowing what information is reliable and credible.

As a person experiencing high blood pressure, you may be skeptical about your condition and the steps to control your blood pressure. As pharmacists, we find various patients battling hypertension, from physically strained workers to mentally stressed office employees. You may also know a relative who must take maintenance medications for their blood pressure. All around us people are trying to manage their blood pressure.

Even famous people like Larry King and Bill Clinton had to spend millions on expensive surgeries and procedures because of high blood pressure and heart complications. Bill Clinton had to lose weight and change his diet to legumes, beans, vegetables, and fruit. CNN interviewer Larry King had a heart attack, causing him to undergo bypass surgery. Blood pressure control is crucial to preventing these complications and procedures.

When you have hypertension, it means the pressure against your blood vessel walls is consistently too high. A blood pressure reading has two numbers: systolic and diastolic pressure. Systolic is the top number which measures blood pressure when the heart is contracting to move blood and diastolic is the bottom number which measures blood pressure when the heart is relaxed and filling with blood. These readings are categorized into ranges indicating whether you have a normal, mild, moderate, or hypertensive crisis, which we will further discuss within the chapters.

Since this disease has no obvious symptoms, many people don't know they have it until the condition has worsened. It is often known as a silent killer. Every individual will experience different symptoms, and most of the time, there are none. High blood pressure can be related to various causes. Nobody is safe from this genetic and lifestyle disease. Nevertheless, proper management and awareness can prevent serious consequences.

You may feel that life dealing with high blood pressure limits you from enjoying your favorite activities. However, many people manage to balance a healthy lifestyle, physical activity, and time with loved ones. You will get results and adapt to your condition with the proper knowledge and consistent effort.

Some patients wait for warning signs before making any changes, which is a dangerous practice. The best way to deal with high blood pressure is early intervention. You may hesitate to get a check-up with your doctor and find out about your results. But the sooner you get the right treatment plan, the better you can prevent further complications from developing. The cost of medications, diet changes, and doctor appointments may seem to be a heavy burden. Nonetheless, the earlier you take that step toward treatment, the less time and money you'll have to waste in the long run.

Different types of treatment plans are available for people with hypertension. Clinical guidelines are followed according to the American College of Cardiology and American Heart's Association (ACC/AHA). The prevalence of high blood pressure in 2015–2018 among adults in the U.S. shows that 116 million people had hypertension. Most of them are recommended medication and still do not have their hypertension under control. This is a great opportunity for education and lifestyle changes.

There are so many risk factors for heart disease and hypertension that affect every household and occupation. Job strain and blood pressure are significantly associated. It is essential to balance your job's physical demands if you have high blood pressure. Having to juggle work, social life, family, and blood pressure may feel overwhelming. You may worry about the sacrifices you have to make and feel impatient about the results.

Hypertension treatment will require you to change your lifestyle, but this does not imply your quality of life will be less. It requires you to make simple changes that give your health a chance, providing you with better opportunities to live fully into your later years. It will be worth all the sacrifices and patience in preventing life-threatening complications. Hypertension is one of the major causes of premature deaths worldwide. Reducing your blood pressure will also prevent other lifestyle diseases since it affects many organs including the heart, brain, and kidneys.

According to the World Health Organization (WHO), 46% of adults worldwide are undiagnosed. Hence, one of the global targets for non-communicable diseases is to reduce their prevalence by 33% between 2010 and 2030. A non-communicable disease is a disease that does not spread from person to person, it is the result of behavior, lifestyle, or genetic factors—not an acute illness.

Some patients with undiagnosed hypertension only learn about their condition after a heart attack resulting from severe hypertension. The risk of heart, brain, and kidney disease will demand more medications, leading to side effects and complications. Fortunately, numerous medications can help you control your hypertension. Although it may take time to find the correct dosage, coordinating with your healthcare professional will make the treatment successful. Moreover, several low-cost yet effective medications have been developed, and health insurance coverage can help you with expenses.

One check-up I witnessed at a clinic was from a patient that seemed physically active and only experienced occasional headaches, dizziness, and fatigue. He seemed like a healthy male in his 50s. He said he went on lengthy bike rides and crash diets to prevent weight gain. However, in between these routines, he would eat fatty foods and drink alcohol. He was surprised to find out that he was experiencing cardiomegaly or heart enlargement. This condition develops when the heart compensates for severe ongoing hypertension.

Another patient had their blood pressure under control after following their prescriptions and lifestyle changes. However, they stopped their medications when they felt their blood pressure was controlled. Some people assume that lifestyle changes are enough to treat all types of hypertension, but you must follow the instructions of your doctor if they advise you to take maintenance medications. Symptoms may return, and your condition may worsen if you stop treatment or return to unhealthy habits.

As previously mentioned, Larry King, a long-time smoker, quit on the day of his heart attack. He has since controlled his risk factors and built The Larry King Cardiac Foundation. David Letterman from *The Late Show*, whose father died of a heart attack, underwent quintuple bypass surgery. He had no complications after surgery and returned to hosting only after six weeks of recovery. These people went through complex procedures and improved their lifestyles. They have since been living their life fully. Many of them actively promote awareness and have supported foundations for cardiovascular diseases.

So how will you effectively monitor and manage your blood pressure? It may be challenging to know when you need to see your doctor. You may need help understanding how to measure your blood pressure initially, but you can get the hang of it quickly with the proper practice and information. Furthermore, automated electronic monitors are available at pharmacies or online. These devices are much easier to use at home to keep track of your numbers.

For every condition, different types of medicines and lifestyle changes can be made. Whatever the cause of your hypertension and the dominant risks in your life, you will find the information you need in this book. It will provide step-by-step guidelines, descriptions, and answers to your questions. We will also debunk some misconceptions about hypertension.

This book will walk you through easily and successfully managing your condition. Learn about your symptoms, medications, lifestyle changes, and other ways to regulate your blood pressure. You will get optimal information and relatable stories from a healthcare provider's perspective translated into simple-to-understand words. Let's get started on your journey to understanding your body and all you need to know about managing high blood pressure.

1

UNDER PRESSURE

D id you know that high blood pressure is a common health concern, even among younger adults? Nearly 1 in 4 adults aged 20 to 44 have high blood pressure, which is a major risk factor for heart attack, stroke, and other serious health problems. Despite the prevalence of high blood pressure in this age group, it is often overlooked and undertreated. Understanding the importance of blood pressure and taking steps to monitor and control it early on can help prevent the development of serious health problems later in life.

OVERVIEW OF BLOOD PRESSURE

We know high blood pressure causes health issues, but what exactly does blood pressure measure? Blood pressure measures the force that moves blood against the walls of your arteries as the heart pumps blood. It is described as having two numbers: systolic and diastolic pressure. When your heart beats, it pumps blood into the circulatory system. Oxygen and nutrients are delivered throughout your body to nourish tissues and organs.

The blood exerts pressure on the arteries by forcing out blood when the heart contracts with every heartbeat. It beats 60 to 100 times a minute, 24 hours a day. The number of times your heart beats in one minute is called a heart rate. Blood pressure differs from heart rate because it measures how powerfully your blood travels through your blood vessels. They are both associated with the heart, but they measure different things. An increased heart rate doesn't mean your blood pressure is also increased.

Blood pressure changes as blood flows through the body. The circulatory system is like a form of plumbing. You could consider the arteries as pipes that follow the basic law of physics. The blood pressure is highest at the start and lowest at the end along smaller branches of arteries. The arteries can also be compared to the physical properties of a garden hose. If you squeeze a hose, the pressure on the walls where you constrict it increases.

The heart creates the maximum pressure for the blood to flow, but the properties of the arteries, such as their elasticity are also important. Hence, the condition of the arteries can affect blood pressure and flow. Moreover, if the arteries narrow, they can block the blood supply to the circulatory system.

If you want to monitor your blood pressure, you should be able to tell the normal blood pressure ranges. National guidelines provide parameters for normal and abnormal blood pressure levels. Blood pressure units are measured in millimeters of mercury or mm Hg. The National Institutes of Health and the American Heart Association (AHA) guidelines set the normal blood pressure below 120 mm Hg systolic and 80 mm Hg diastolic. Just remember, normal blood pressure is 120/80!

However, these guidelines have changed over the years. The older guidelines from 2003 were updated in 2017 and are currently being used. Since AHA followed the 2017 guidelines, it has allowed earlier intervention for people with high blood pressure.

Before the update, a prehypertension category existed between 120–139/80–89 mm Hg. Now, it is referred to as elevated blood pressure between 120–129/<80 mm Hg. People at risk of hypertension and in the earlier stages of hypertension are recommended lifestyle modifications. Moreover, people with 130–139 mm Hg/80–89 mm Hg qualify as stage 1 hypertension.

The numbers seem confusing at first, but with practice and guidance from your healthcare provider, you can get the hang of it. Blood pressure fluctuates based on different factors. Your blood pressure increases when you jog or ride a roller coaster. Yet, your blood pressure is lower when lying down or spending a day at the spa. Even age, medications, and changes in position affect your blood pressure. That's why there are certain guidelines followed when reading your blood pressure.

You may wonder why you need to know your blood pressure. When you get a check-up or go to a hospital, a healthcare provider will most likely ask for a reading. Blood pressure is the most commonly measured clinical parameter because it is a major determinant for diagnosis and treatment. Checking your blood pressure at every doctor visit allows for early detection and intervention to prevent further complications. This is especially important in those patients without symptoms of high blood pressure.

PHYSIOLOGY OF BLOOD PRESSURE REGULATION

Blood pressure regulation is a complex process that is operated by several mechanisms all at once. It gives insight into the working of the heart and vessels. If your body fails to regulate its blood pressure, it becomes too high or too low. This can lead to a wide range of diseases. This regulation mechanism is very important to maintaining healthy blood pressure to provide all organs with adequate blood supply and eliminate necessary waste.

Blood that gets delivered to the body picks up waste products and toxins. It regulates temperature and carries defending cells to tissue damage. Your heart, kidneys, and brain can become damaged if you have high blood pressure and your blood circulation does not function properly. High blood pressure is a major risk for complications and even fatal diseases.

Short-term adaptation and long-term maintenance of blood pressure are needed to keep it within a normal range. When your blood pressure needs rapid adjustments, it is regulated by a baroreceptor reflex. This reflex is a short-term regulation mechanism that influences the nervous (nerves) and endocrine (hormones) systems.

Higher blood pressure increases the activity of these baroreceptors. This increase reduces heart rate and the widening of blood vessels and arteries in order to lower blood pressure. However, when blood pressure decreases, receptor activity becomes lower. This reduction leads to an increased heart rate and vasoconstriction or narrowing of passages in order to raise blood pressure. These reactions adjust the blood pressure accordingly to keep it in the normal range.

The blood pressure regulation system keeps your blood pressure in a healthy range. Your heart, nervous system, hormones, and kidneys interact through the blood pressure regulation system. Your heart and kidneys work together and can affect each other's conditions. Therefore, if you have kidney disease, it can lead to heart disease and vice versa. In fact, they share many risk factors, such as diabetes and high blood pressure.

The heart pumps blood through your blood vessels, and the force of blood flow against the vessel walls is your blood pressure. The kidneys cleanse your blood and remove excess salt and water. This role makes it an important factor in regulating your blood pressure. It also helps control your blood volume and the diameter of blood vessels.

The kidney's other roles affecting blood pressure are regulating electrolytes and producing hormones.

Without the kidneys, your blood would have too much waste and water. Without the heart, your kidneys won't have enough blood that delivers oxygen for them to function.

The impact of high blood pressure on the kidney is by constant stretching of small blood vessels in the kidney's tubules. The repeated stress on the vessel walls can cause scarring, leading to kidney problems. People with kidney disease fail to use the renin-angiotensin-aldosterone system (RAAS) system for blood regulation.

RAAS is a hormone system that can help regulate blood pressure and volume. Compared to the baroreceptor reflex, RAAS is slower but a long-term means of regulating blood pressure. The RAAS system relies on several hormones to increase blood volume and peripheral resistance. This resistance is used to create blood pressure and blood flow. When blood vessels constrict (vasoconstriction), it increases peripheral resistance—when blood vessels dilate (vasodilation), peripheral resistance decreases, and so does blood pressure.

When your blood pressure drops, the kidney secretes an enzyme called renin into the bloodstream. It is released when there is more salt in the blood, less blood flow in the kidney, or through the sympathetic nervous system. Renin is responsible for producing the angiotensin II hormone.

Angiotensin II causes vasoconstriction. Hence, the increase in angiotensin II can cause high blood pressure. Angiotensin II goes through different conversions, which starts off as angiotensinogen. Renin converts angiotensinogen to angiotensin I, eventually converted by the angiotensinogen-converting enzyme (ACE) into angiotensin II.

The names and terms may sound confusing, but you don't have to memorize them. Being familiar with and understanding how your body works can help you understand your condition and the medications you may use for treatment.

These processes create different responses that alter blood pressure. ACE, primarily from the lungs, also gets rid of bradykinin. Bradykinin is a vasodilator, which means it can widen the passage of blood. If it gets reduced, this leads to vasoconstriction or narrowing of passages.

Angiotensin II hormone will boost the release of the aldosterone hormone. Aldosterone will make the kidneys retain more salt and water, which results in more plasma volume and arterial pressure. Another way angiotensin II can increase plasma volume is through thirst and the antidiuretic hormone (ADH).

Aldosterone increases sodium while decreasing potassium and hydrogen through secretion in the kidneys. Since it can increase blood pressure through this process, several anti-hypertensive medications act through aldosterone.

This sequence of reactions is called the RAAS system. It efficiently and quickly increases blood pressure to maintain proper blood flow to vital organs. Since the RAAS system can increase blood volume and pressure, it can cause complications in certain individuals if it becomes overactive.

The cardiac cycle empties blood into the arterioles at an even rate, but the blood pressure undergoes natural variations from one heartbeat to another. Blood pressure changes in response to stress, nutritional factors, drugs, diseases, or position. The body regulates blood pressure by changes in response to the cardiac output and stroke volume.

When you suddenly stand up after lying down, your blood pressure temporarily increases. This rise ensures enough blood and oxygen gets to your brain. Changing positions can certainly impact your blood pressure.

When lying down, your heart doesn't have to pump so hard to circulate blood throughout your body. Most of your body parts are at the same level as your heart, which explains why you have lower blood pressure. Although minor changes in blood pressure exist, there is no medical consensus on the difference between positions.

A noticeable change in blood pressure is from lying down to standing up. Standing up causes the blood to pool in your lower body. Hence your blood pressure temporarily drops. This drop adjusts your body by making your heart beat faster to pump more blood, increasing your blood pressure. Occasionally you may feel this sudden drop in blood pressure when going to a standing position; this is called orthostatic hypotension.

Your blood pressure increases during exercise to help deliver more oxygen and nutrients to your muscles. This rise is usually temporary. Your blood pressure should gradually return to normal after exercise. During exercise, your systolic blood pressure increases more than diastolic. Your heart pumps harder and faster to circulate blood to the muscles. Since systolic represents the pressure when your heart beats and diastolic is when the heart rests, it may be concerning if the diastolic blood pressure significantly increases after exercising.

During exercise, your systolic blood pressure may rise between 160 and 220 mm Hg. Anywhere higher than 200 mm Hg should be discussed with a healthcare provider. A person with systolic blood pressure up to 250 mm Hg is considered to have exercise hypertension. Nevertheless, factors such as diet, drugs, and medical conditions may also affect how your heart responds to exercise.

Cardiac output, or the volume of blood pumped by the heart per minute, increases through an increased heart rate. This also happens when exercising. The blood vessels relax and widen during heavy exertion, offsetting the increased heart rate. This process regulates the amount of blood and oxygen going to your muscles. However, blood vessels narrow down when stressed, increasing blood pressure.

Your blood pressure fluctuates as a compensatory mechanism to help your body function properly. Blood pressure regulation has to maintain a high enough pressure that allows for blood flow to the organs and tissues but not too high that it causes harm. When your body goes through chronic hypertension, you can't pinpoint an exact cause. Rather, it is a consequence of the interaction of multiple risk factors.

Healthy arteries are smooth, and blood passes through easily. However, fats, cholesterol, and calcium can build up in the inner walls. This buildup, called plaque, slows blood flow, or may even block it. Blockages like plaque can make blood vessels too narrow and hardened to function properly. Blood pressure increases to compensate for this problem. Pressure increases to help push blood through the vessels, delivering proper blood flow to organs. However, it can lead to serious health problems if your body constantly compensates for different issues that affect your blood pressure.

There are no obvious symptoms at first, but they can develop as plaque builds up in the arteries. Usual signs are chest discomfort, dizziness, or excessive sweating. Since there is less blood supply to the legs and arms, it may cause pain and difficulty walking. Moreover, blocked arteries can lead to hypertension, stroke, or death. These serious consequences show us why it is so important to monitor your blood pressure and maintain a healthy lifestyle.

AN OVERWORKED HEART: THE DEFINITION AND CAUSES OF HIGH BLOOD PRESSURE

Hypertension is a medical term for chronic high blood pressure. High blood pressure or hypertension is when the force of blood pushing through your vessels is consistently too high. Blood vessels or arteries create resistance to blood flow when they become narrow. This effect leads to higher blood pressure.

Nearly half of American adults could be diagnosed with hypertension. It gradually develops over several years without being noticed. However, even without symptoms, hypertension can cause serious damage if left untreated. Early detection can be done with regular blood pressure readings. It is important to understand your blood pressure readings. Your doctor may ask you to check your blood pressure over a span of a few weeks or daily—depending on your condition.

High blood pressure causes damage to your tissues and organs. It starts in your arteries and heart. Your hypertension causes harm by increasing the workload of the heart and blood vessels, making them less efficient. This effect gradually damages the inner walls of the arteries. If the damage is prolonged, your hypertension worsens, leading to other harmful diseases.

Your blood pressure reading consists of two numbers. The top number is the systolic pressure when your heart beats and pumps blood. The bottom number is the diastolic pressure when your heart rests between beats.

There are currently five categories that define blood pressure readings.

- **Healthy** – comes in a blood pressure reading of less than 120/80 mm Hg.
- **Elevated** – is between 120–129 mm Hg for the top number and less than 80 mm Hg for the bottom number. Lifestyle changes are recommended for this category.
- **Stage 1 hypertension** – has a systolic pressure between 130–139 mm Hg and a diastolic pressure between 80–89 mm Hg.
- **Stage 2 hypertension** – has a reading equal to or higher than 140/90 mm Hg.
- **Hypertensive crisis** – is when your reading is over 180/120 mm Hg. Blood pressure within these numbers means you need urgent medical attention.

There are also different types of hypertension, called primary and secondary hypertension. They both result from high blood pressure. The difference between the two is the causes related to each. Primary hypertension doesn't have a conclusive or known cause, while secondary hypertension does. Nevertheless, they both lead to serious consequences if untreated.

There are key differences between the two. Primary hypertension occurs more often than secondary hypertension. Various risk factors increase your chances of developing it over the years. Unlike primary hypertension, secondary hypertension is rare and sudden. Moreover, it is caused by underlying conditions. The treatment plan for both may be taken with a different approach by your healthcare provider. Regardless, a healthy lifestyle is vital for both.

Primary Hypertension

Primary hypertension is also known as idiopathic or essential hypertension. It is a type of hypertension with multiple factors and doesn't have one distinct cause. The majority of people with high blood pressure have this type of hypertension. It is considered primary hypertension if none of the underlying causes of secondary hypertension exists. Your doctor will review your medical history and medications to rule this out.

According to the World Health Organization, 90–95% of adults have primary hypertension. It gradually develops through the years due to various factors. Since primary hypertension is not due to another medical condition, many causes are considered to manage it.

Risk factors include:

- Age (common in ages 65 years and older)
- Family history or genes
- Race
- Diet (high-salt intake)
- Obesity or being overweight
- Sedentary lifestyle or being inactive
- Stress
- Alcohol consumption
- Cigarette use

Secondary Hypertension

Secondary hypertension develops from an underlying condition, disease, or medication side effect. When high blood pressure is caused by a direct or distinct condition, it is considered secondary hypertension. According to the National Institute of Health, this rare type of hypertension occurs only in 2–10% of people with chronic high blood pressure. It is also known as resistant hypertension.

Common causes that are associated with it are:

- Kidney disease (damage to the kidneys can trigger the production of renin)
- Thyroid disease

- Adrenal disease (it causes hormone imbalance)
- Obstructive sleep apnea
- Oral contraceptives or birth control pills
- Nonsteroidal anti-inflammatory drugs (NSAIDs such as aspirin or ibuprofen)
- Antidepressants
- Decongestants
- Stimulants

Both primary and secondary hypertension usually occurs without specific symptoms. However, there are some indications of secondary hypertension, including the following:

- You are resistant to blood pressure medications, or they stop being effective.
- You develop hypertension suddenly with abrupt symptoms.
- Low potassium and high calcium levels.
- High creatinine levels.
- If you are at low risk but your blood pressure is too high. Nevertheless, people that are at high risk may still develop high blood pressure through secondary hypertension.

Primary and secondary hypertension can both exist when there is a sudden worsening of blood pressure. If a secondary cause is considered, additional tests such as kidney and heart ultrasound, electrocardiogram, and cholesterol screening may be conducted by your doctor. Physical signs indicating secondary hypertension include weight changes, swelling, abnormal hair growth, and stretch marks around the abdomen.

Moreover, secondary hypertension treatment options focus on the underlying issues diagnosed, such as kidney problems. If it is caused by a medication, an alternative may be recommended. Secondary hypertension has a positive outlook with treatment, especially if detected early. It will only last as long as you have the secondary condition.

Most cases of hypertension typically have no symptoms, even if your blood pressure becomes dangerously high. This is why it is often called a silent killer. It may cause damage to the body without you realizing it until your condition is severe or a heart attack occurs. Moreover, you can have high blood pressure for years without symptoms. It quietly causes damage that threatens your life.

A few people who experience symptoms may have headaches, shortness of breath, or nosebleeds. Nevertheless, the symptoms that take place will vary. They aren't specific and occur when your high blood pressure is at a life-threatening stage. According to the

American Heart Association, nosebleeds and headaches don't happen until someone is in a hypertensive crisis.

Since many people are unaware that they have uncontrolled blood pressure, it is important to get regular blood pressure checks from a healthcare provider. When you visit a hospital or your doctor, they will get your blood pressure reading first. This is to ensure that it is within a healthy range. It also helps catch any potential issues early on.

Annual physicals and preventive maintenance are important for monitoring blood pressure. It can help detect and address potential problems before they become more serious. Your healthcare provider can discuss your risks and other readings to help monitor your blood pressure.

Hypertension can cause various damages to the body. Complications with your organs and other body functions will interfere with your quality of life. The damage high blood pressure can inflict may lead to life-threatening complications. It often has a domino effect of consequences on your health. High blood pressure can lead to the following:

Damage to the heart and arteries

High blood pressure causes strain on the heart, leading to enlargement and other issues. It increases the workload on your circulatory system, failing to supply blood efficiently. Arteries should be flexible, strong, and elastic, while blood is supposed to flow smoothly through the arteries. It should efficiently supply nutrients and oxygen to your body.

- Heart attack – high blood pressure narrows and stiffens the arteries, which increases the risk of a heart attack.
- Heart failure – the strain on the heart can cause the heart muscle to weaken and fail.
- Coronary artery disease – when the blood supply to the heart is affected by decreased blood flow, it leads to chest pain (angina) or irregular heart rhythms (arrhythmias).
- Peripheral artery disease (PAD) – damaged arteries can lead to atherosclerosis. This condition limits blood flow to the legs, arms, stomach, and head, causing pain or fatigue.
- Damaged and narrowed arteries – damaged arteries can collect fats or plaque, making the artery walls narrow and hardened.
- Aneurysm – it is when a section of an artery wall becomes enlarged and forms a bulge. This bulge or aneurysm can rupture and cause internal bleeding.

Damage to the brain

The brain needs blood and oxygen supply to function properly. High blood pressure and heart problems can cause life-threatening brain damage.

- Stroke – if your hypertension worsens, blood vessels in the brain are damaged. The clogged blood vessels in the brain block blood flow, leading to stroke.
- Transient ischemic attack (TIA) – it is sometimes called a ministroke, which is also a warning sign for a full-blown stroke. TIA is a brief, temporary interruption of blood supply to the brain due to hardened arteries or blood clots.
- Dementia – when the blood flow to the brain is limited, it leads to vascular dementia.
- Mild cognitive impairment – this is the transition between the normal part of aging and dementia, which affects understanding and memory.

Damage to the kidneys

Hypertension affects the crucial role of the kidney in filtering blood, which requires healthy blood vessels.

- Kidney scarring – is when tiny blood vessels linked to the kidney become scarred, leading to kidney failure. It is also known as glomerulosclerosis.
- Kidney failure – high blood pressure can damage the arteries in the kidneys. When blood isn't filtered properly, dangerous levels of fluid and waste accumulate in the blood.

Damage to the eyes

The eyes have tiny, delicate blood vessels. If these vessels are strained or damaged, the following may occur:

- Retinopathy – is caused by damaged blood vessels in the retina. The retina is the light-sensitive tissue at the back of your eyes. This can lead to bleeding, blurred vision, and total vision loss.

- Choroidopathy – is the fluid buildup under the retina, causing distorted vision. It can also cause scarring.
- Optic neuropathy – it is also known as nerve damage. The optic nerve can be damaged when blood flow is blocked, leading to bleeding and vision loss.

Sexual dysfunction

Hypertension can reduce blood flow to the body, including the genitals. Their function is impaired due to limited blood flow and oxygen.

- Erectile dysfunction – men may have difficulty maintaining or having an erection as they age. High blood pressure increases their risk of experiencing this.
- Lower libido – women may experience a decreased sex drive, vaginal dryness, and difficulty having an orgasm.

The prevalence of hypertension per age group

The prevalence of hypertension is a major public health challenge in the United States because of its consequences on people's quality of life. The number of adults with hypertension in 2015–2016 was 29%. This increases with age, as it is a risk factor for high blood pressure. There were 7.5% of adults between 18–39 who had hypertension. For ages 40–59, it hiked to 33.2%. Lastly, those aged 60 and over had a 63.1% prevalence of hypertension.

MEASURING AND DIAGNOSING

Measuring your blood pressure is an important routine that you should learn. Consistently monitoring it helps you control your blood pressure. You can ask a family member to help you keep track. We often find older people who repeatedly measure their blood pressure when they feel distressed. Most often, it is better to calm them down before taking that reading. The following information will guide you in measuring someone else's or your own blood pressure:

A blood pressure reading is taken with a cuff or a sphygmomanometer. This strap-like device is used by your doctor for a more accurate reading.

A blood pressure reading tests the force exerted on the arteries. It is measured in millimeters of mercury (mm Hg), including the below two readings:

- Systolic blood pressure is found first or at the top of the denomination. Systolic pressure is the force inside the artery walls as the heart beats.
- Diastolic blood pressure is the second or lower denomination in a blood pressure reading. Diastolic pressure is when the heart is at rest.

A blood pressure measurement can be used to diagnose hypertension in its early stages. High blood pressure usually doesn't have warning signs or symptoms, so regularly measuring your blood pressure helps you get treated early.

It is the primary test for screening hypertension in a patient. A blood pressure measurement is often required when you get a regular check-up at your doctor or the hospital. It is recommended that adults have their blood pressure tested every few years or yearly if they are at risk.

You may be familiar with these steps in measuring blood pressure if you've been to the hospital or for a health check-up:

- A nurse or healthcare provider will ask you to sit in a chair with your feet flat on the ground.
- Your arm should rest on a table at your heart's level.
- The blood pressure cuff is wrapped around your upper arm to fit just right, with the bottom edge of the cuff placed just above your elbow.
- Using a small hand pump or a button, the cuff wrapped around your arm will be inflated.

- If a manual blood pressure cuff is used, your healthcare provider will use a stethoscope to listen to your blood flow and pulse.
- While the cuff inflates, it will tighten around your arm. And as it deflates, the blood pressure falls.
- When the blood pressure falls, the sound of blood pulsing is first heard. This is recorded as systolic pressure.
- The blood pulsing sound disappears, and the cuff's air is released. Once the sound completely stops, it is recorded as diastolic pressure.
- An automated device will display a digital reading after inflating and deflating on its own.

Your blood pressure may be slightly affected by factors such as medications, caffeine, physical activity, emotional state, and the time of the day. Nevertheless, there are no preparations before taking your blood pressure. It is recommended to monitor your blood pressure frequently, particularly in the morning as you wake up.

After taking your blood pressure, you must record your results. This will contain your systolic and diastolic pressure. You can check the chart for the categories of hypertension to determine if your blood pressure is under control. Your doctor will provide a diagnosis and treatment plan based on your blood pressure readings. If you track your blood pressure at home, it is good practice to keep a notebook to log your readings and bring them to your visits with your physician or pharmacist.

A diagnosis of elevated blood pressure is determined with two or more blood pressure readings. They may recommend home monitoring with an automated blood pressure device. However, you will still be required to visit your doctor regularly. Monitoring your blood pressure will help update or optimize your treatment.

If you suspect you or a family member has high blood pressure, an appointment with a doctor should be scheduled. Testing your blood pressure only takes a few minutes. A blood pressure screening is a painless procedure. However, some other tests and procedures may be requested. Your doctor will check for causes of high blood pressure and assess the risk from the condition or the treatment. Procedures and tests included in the diagnosis are:

- Blood tests or complete blood count (CBC)

    o Electrolytes
    o Blood urea nitrogen (BUN)
    o Creatinine levels (to assess kidney issues)

- Lipid profile for cholesterol
- Glucose test for blood sugar
- Special tests for hormones (to assess adrenal or thyroid issues)
- Urine tests for electrolytes and hormones
- Eye examination with an ophthalmoscope (to assess ocular damage)
- Ultrasound of kidneys
- CT scan of the abdomen

For people with severe hypertension, damage to the heart or blood vessels should be determined with the following tests:

- Electrocardiogram (ECG) – detects the electrical activity of the heart. ECG evaluates the damage to the heart muscles.
- Echocardiogram – an ultrasound examination of the heart through the chest. An echocardiogram will detect abnormalities in your heart size, heart wall, heart valve, and

blood clots. Moreover, it can measure the strength of the heart muscle. It is more comprehensive than ECG but also costly.

- Chest X-ray – a simple procedure that provides an estimated heart size.
- Doppler ultrasound – checks the blood flow through the arteries in your arms, legs, hands, and feet. It detects peripheral vascular disease caused by the narrowing of arteries.

Since hypertension usually doesn't have symptoms, your doctor will ask about your medical records, current medications, family history, vices, and other risk factors. In addition, a physical exam is conducted using a stethoscope. In addition, your doctor will listen to your heartbeat for any abnormalities. They may also check for your pulse to see if they are weak or absent.

Now that you have a solid understanding of blood pressure and hypertension, it's important to dive deeper into the risk factors contributing to developing high blood pressure.

2

WHAT PUTS YOU AT RISK FOR HIGH BLOOD PRESSURE?

D id you know that hypertension impacts over 30% of the global adult population, affecting more than one billion individuals? It serves as the primary risk factor for various cardiovascular conditions, including coronary heart disease and stroke, as well as chronic kidney disease, heart failure, arrhythmia, and dementia.

In this chapter, I will be walking you through the risk factors associated with hypertension. Read on to find out how you, or somebody you care about, could be harboring habits that are impacting their health.

RISK FACTORS FOR HIGH BLOOD PRESSURE

Understanding the risk factors for high blood pressure is essential for effective prevention and management of hypertension. Various factors contribute to an individual's risk of developing high blood pressure, including age, gender, genetics, and lifestyle choices. By gaining a deeper understanding of these risk factors, individuals can make informed decisions to minimize their risk and maintain optimal cardiovascular health.

1. Age: The risk of developing high blood pressure increases as we age. With time, blood vessels can lose their elasticity, which can contribute to increased resistance and higher blood pressure levels. According to the American Heart Association, nearly two-thirds of adults over 60 years old have high blood pressure. However, younger individuals are not immune to hypertension, and it is essential to monitor blood pressure levels and adopt healthy lifestyle habits early in life.

2. Gender: There are differences in the prevalence of high blood pressure between men and women. Men are generally more likely to develop hypertension at a younger age, while women's risk increases significantly after menopause. Estrogen is believed to play a protective role against hypertension in premenopausal women, but this protection diminishes with age. Regardless of gender, it is crucial to be proactive about blood pressure management and adopt lifestyle changes that promote heart health.

3. Genetics: Family history and genetics can significantly influence an individual's risk of developing high blood pressure. If one or both of your parents have hypertension, your risk of developing the condition is higher. Although you cannot change your genetic predisposition, understanding your family history can help you make more informed decisions about your lifestyle and healthcare to mitigate your risk.

4. Lifestyle factors: A wide range of lifestyle factors can contribute to high blood pressure, including:

a. **Poor diet**: Consuming a diet high in salt, saturated fats, and processed foods can increase blood pressure levels. Adopting a heart-healthy diet, such as the DASH (Dietary Approaches to Stop Hypertension) diet, which emphasizes whole grains, fruits, vegetables, lean proteins, and low-fat dairy products, can help lower blood pressure, and maintain optimal cardiovascular health.

b. **Physical inactivity**: Leading a sedentary lifestyle can contribute to weight gain, decreased cardiovascular fitness, and increased blood pressure levels. Engaging in regular physical activity, such as walking, swimming, or cycling, can help lower blood pressure, improve heart health, and promote overall well-being.

c. **Excessive alcohol consumption:** Drinking alcohol in moderation (one drink per day for women and up to two drinks per day for men) may have some cardiovascular benefits. However, excessive alcohol consumption can lead to weight gain, liver damage, and increased blood pressure levels. Limiting alcohol intake can help prevent hypertension and promote better overall health.

d. **Stress**: Chronic stress can elevate blood pressure levels by causing the release of stress hormones, which can constrict blood vessels and increase heart rate. Developing effective stress management techniques, such as deep breathing exercises, meditation, and yoga, and engaging in hobbies or activities that promote relaxation and enjoyment, can help manage blood pressure and promote overall well-being.

Apart from these, obesity, a sedentary lifestyle, tobacco use, smoking, and certain medical conditions are all significant risk factors as well. Let's delve deeper into these risk factors and their impact on hypertension:

1. Obesity: Excess body weight, particularly around the abdomen, increases the risk of high blood pressure. Obesity can cause the heart to work harder to pump blood, leading to increased pressure on the arterial walls. Additionally, obesity is often associated with other health issues such as sleep apnea, diabetes, and high cholesterol, which can further contribute to hypertension. Implementing a weight loss plan through healthy dietary changes and regular physical activity can help lower blood pressure and reduce the risk of complications.

2. Sedentary lifestyle: A lack of physical activity can lead to weight gain and decreased cardiovascular fitness, both of which contribute to high blood pressure. Physical inactivity may also result in the weakening of the heart muscle, which can lead to a less efficient pumping action and elevated blood pressure. Incorporating regular exercise into your daily routine can improve heart health, lower blood pressure, and promote overall well-being.

3. Tobacco use: Tobacco use, including smoking and smokeless tobacco products, can cause a temporary increase in blood pressure and damage the cardiovascular system over time. The chemicals found in tobacco can narrow blood vessels and increase arterial stiffness, leading to elevated blood pressure levels. Quitting tobacco use and avoiding exposure to secondhand smoke can significantly reduce the risk of hypertension and its associated complications.

4. Smoking: Similar to tobacco use, smoking can cause both short-term and long-term increases in blood pressure. The nicotine in cigarettes can constrict blood vessels, increase heart rate, and elevate blood pressure temporarily. Over time, smoking can damage blood vessels and contribute to the development of atherosclerosis, further increasing the risk of hypertension. Quitting smoking is one of the most effective ways to lower blood pressure and improve cardiovascular health.

5. Sleep apnea: Sleep apnea is a medical condition characterized by repeated interruptions in breathing during sleep, leading to decreased oxygen levels in the blood. This can cause the release of stress hormones, increased heart rate, and elevated blood pressure. Treating sleep apnea with continuous positive airway pressure (CPAP) therapy or other appropriate interventions can help lower blood pressure and reduce the risk of hypertension-related complications.

6. Kidney disease: The kidneys play a crucial role in regulating blood pressure by filtering blood and removing excess salt and water. When the kidneys are damaged or not functioning properly, they may be unable to remove excess salt and water effectively, leading to increased blood volume and elevated blood pressure. Proper management of kidney disease, including medication and lifestyle changes, can help control blood pressure and prevent further kidney damage.

7. **Diabetes**: Individuals with diabetes are at a higher risk of developing high blood pressure due to the effects of high blood sugar levels on blood vessels and the kidneys. Over time, elevated blood sugar can damage blood vessels, making them less flexible and more prone to narrowing, leading to increased blood pressure. Additionally, diabetes can impact kidney function, further contributing to hypertension. Managing diabetes through medication, diet, and exercise is essential for maintaining healthy blood pressure levels and preventing complications.

Understanding and addressing these risk factors can significantly reduce an individual's risk of developing high blood pressure and its associated complications. By adopting a healthy lifestyle, staying physically active, maintaining a balanced diet, managing stress, and limiting alcohol intake, individuals can effectively manage their blood pressure levels and improve their overall cardiovascular health.

In essence, taking control of one's lifestyle and under-standing the various risk factors for high blood pres-sure is critical for effective prevention and management of hypertension. By making informed decisions about diet, exercise, stress management, and other lifestyle factors, individuals can reduce their risk of developing high blood pressure and maintain optimal cardiovascular health. Regular check-ups with a healthcare provider can also help identify any poten-tial issues early on and ensure that appropriate inter-ventions are implemented to maintain healthy blood pressure.

SUPPORTING FACTORS

Environmental factors can also contribute to the devel-opment of high blood pressure, including stress, certain medications, and pregnancy. Understanding the impact of these factors on blood pressure levels is essential for effective management and prevention of hypertension.

1. Stress: Chronic stress can have a significant impact on blood pressure by causing the release of stress hormones, which can constrict blood vessels and increase heart rate. While short-term stress may lead to temporary spikes in blood pressure, long-term stress can contribute to sustained hypertension. It is impor-tant to identify and manage stressors in one's life to maintain healthy blood pressure levels.

2. Medication: Certain medications can contribute to high blood pressure, either as a direct side effect or through interactions with other medications or substances. Common medications that may affect blood pressure include decongestants, nonsteroidal anti-inflammatory drugs (NSAIDs), oral contraceptives, and certain antidepressants. It is crucial to discuss potential side effects and interactions with your healthcare provider before starting any new medication and to monitor your blood pressure closely while taking medications that may impact it. If you suspect that a medication may be contributing to your high blood pressure, speak with your healthcare provider about possible alternatives or adjustments to your treatment plan.

3. Pregnancy: High blood pressure can develop during pregnancy, either as a pre-existing condition (chronic hypertension) or as a pregnancy-related complication (gestational hypertension or preeclampsia). Pregnant women with high blood pressure are at an increased risk of complications for both themselves and their babies, including preterm birth, low birth weight, and placental abruption. It is essential for women with high blood pressure to receive appropriate prenatal care and work closely with their healthcare providers to monitor and manage their blood pressure throughout pregnancy. In some cases, medication may be prescribed to help control blood pressure levels, while in others, lifestyle changes, such as dietary modifications and exercise may be recommended.

4. Environmental factors: Exposure to certain environmental factors, such as air pollution and noise pollution, has been linked to increased blood pressure levels. Long-term exposure to air pollution, particularly particulate matter, can cause inflammation and oxidative stress, leading to blood vessel damage and elevated blood pressure. Similarly, chronic exposure to high noise levels, especially during nighttime, can contribute to stress and disrupt sleep patterns, both of which can impact blood pressure. To minimize the effects of these environmental factors on blood pressure, consider using air purifiers, noise-canceling headphones, or other strategies to reduce exposure to air and noise pollution.

Remember, understanding blood pressure, its risk factors, and the role of environmental factors is crucial in managing hypertension effectively. By adopting a healthy lifestyle, addressing potential risk factors, and staying vigilant about the impact of stress, medication, and pregnancy on blood pressure levels, individuals can significantly reduce their risk of developing high blood pressure and its associated complications.

In the next chapter, we will explore various medications and strategies to avoid potential interactions with other drugs or supplements. Staying informed and working closely with your healthcare provider will empower you to find the best treatment plan to manage your high blood pressure and enhance your overall well-being.

3

MEDICATIONS FOR MANAGING HIGH BLOOD PRESSURE

A s we embark on this new chapter of our journey together, I'd like to take a moment to discuss the diverse range of medications available for managing high blood pressure and offer some guidance on steering clear of harmful drug interactions. You might be surprised to learn that the simultaneous use of multiple medications, a phenomenon referred to as polypharmacy, can significantly increase the likelihood of experiencing adverse reactions.

It's a curious fact that the more medications we introduce into our systems, the greater the chances of encountering harmful drug interactions. Studies have demonstrated that patients who take between five and nine medications face a 50% probability of experiencing an adverse drug interaction. Even more staggering is that this risk skyrockets to a complete 100% when an individual takes twenty or more medications concurrently.

Moreover, as stated by Health Research Funding, almost 30% of all hospital admissions can be attributed to polypharmacy, making it the fifth leading cause of death in the United States. That's correct—the excessive consumption of medications can pose a severe and potentially fatal risk to our well-being.

As we delve deeper into this chapter, I aim to provide original, insightful information on managing high blood pressure through various medications. Remember the importance of vigilance and caution when avoiding the dangerous territory of harmful drug interactions.

Medications undoubtedly play a vital role in the quest to manage high blood pressure, a widespread and potentially severe health concern. High blood pressure, if left unaddressed, can lead to various complications, such as heart disease, stroke, and kidney failure. Identifying the most effective medications to control this condition is important.

Various medications are available for treating high blood pressure, each working through distinct mechanisms to maintain healthy blood pressure levels. Some of these medications function by reducing fluid volume within the body, thereby lessening the pressure exerted on blood vessels. Others operate by relaxing the blood vessels, enabling smoother blood flow, and reducing pressure. Yet another category of high blood pressure medications targets specific hormones that contribute to elevated blood pressure, effectively blocking their impact.

Collaborating closely with a healthcare provider is essential to ascertain the most suitable medication or combination of medications tailored to an individual's unique needs. Medical professionals possess the necessary expertise to assess each patient's medical history, current health condition, and other factors that may influence the choice of medication. It is crucial to remember that managing high blood pressure is not a one-size-fits-all approach, and a healthcare provider can help determine the most effective treatment plan for each person.

Once the appropriate medication or combination of medications has been prescribed, it is important to follow the healthcare provider's instructions closely. This includes taking the medications as prescribed, adhering to the recommended dosages, and maintaining a consistent schedule. Deviating from the prescribed regimen may reduce effectiveness and potentially exacerbate the underlying condition.

In addition to following the prescribed treatment plan, monitoring any potential side effects or interactions with other medications is crucial. As discussed earlier, the risk of harmful drug interactions increases with the number of medications being taken concurrently. Consequently, it is vital to maintain open communication with your healthcare provider about all medications you are currently taking, including over-the-counter drugs, supplements, and herbal remedies. This will enable the healthcare provider to evaluate the potential for interactions and adjust the medication regimen if necessary.

Furthermore, being proactive in identifying and reporting any side effects that may arise while taking high blood pressure medications is essential. Some side effects might be temporary and resolved independently, while others could be more serious and require medical intervention. By closely monitoring your body's response to the medications, you can help your health-care provider make informed decisions about your treatment plan and ensure your safety and well-being.

HOW DO BLOOD PRESSURE MEDICINES WORK?

Blood pressure medicines, known as antihypertensives, are designed to regulate and lower high blood pressure. These medications function through various mechanisms, targeting different aspects of the cardiovascular system to maintain healthy blood pressure. Here are some of the primary ways in which these medicines work:

1. **Diuretics**: These medications, sometimes called "water pills," aid the kidneys in removing excess sodium and water from the body. This fluid volume reduction decreases blood vessel pressure, ultimately lowering blood pressure.
2. **Beta-blockers**: By blocking the effects of the hormone epinephrine, also known as adrenaline, beta-blockers help slow down the heart rate and reduce the force with which the heart pumps blood. This results in decreased blood pressure.
3. **Calcium channel blockers**: These medications inhibit the movement of calcium into the muscle cells of the heart and blood vessels. This action relaxes the blood vessels and reduces the

force of the heart's contractions, leading to a decline in blood pressure.

4. **ACE inhibitors**: Angiotensin-converting enzyme (ACE) inhibitors prevent the production of angiotensin II, a hormone that causes blood vessels to constrict. ACE inhibitors promote the relaxation of blood vessels by inhibiting this hormone and effectively lowering blood pressure. Remember the RAAS system from earlier?

5. **Angiotensin II receptor blockers (ARBs)**: Similar to ACE inhibitors, ARBs block the action of angiotensin II but do so by preventing it from binding to its receptors. This interference results in relaxed blood vessels and decreased blood pressure.

6. **Alpha-blockers**: Alpha-blockers relax blood vessels to reduce resistance in blood flow.

7. **Alpha-beta blockers**: Combined alpha-beta blockers are often used in hypertensive crises and are given through an IV drip. They also have an oral form used in patients who are at risk for heart failure or in pregnancy.

8. **Central-acting agents**: Central agonists reduce tension in the blood vessels.

9. **Vasodilators**: Blood vessel dilators relax the

muscle in the blood vessel wall, allowing the vessels to widen and improve blood flow.

10. **Aldosterone receptor antagonists**: ARAs inhibit the hormone aldosterone and promote the excretion of sodium and water and the retention of potassium, helping to reduce blood volume and lowering blood pressure.

11. **Direct renin inhibitors**: Directly inhibiting renin, an enzyme that triggers a sequence of reactions leading to blood vessel constriction and sodium retention, helps relax blood vessels, and reduces fluid retention.

WHAT ARE THE BENEFITS AND RISKS OF BLOOD PRESSURE MEDICINES?

In this section, I will walk you through the benefits of blood pressure medications. Read on to find out more.

Benefits:

1. High blood pressure, if left untreated, can lead to several severe health issues, such as heart attack, stroke, kidney disease, and vision loss. Blood pressure medicines help minimize the risk of these complications by effectively managing the condition.

2. Properly controlled blood pressure enables individuals to lead healthier and more active lives without the constant worry of potential complications arising from elevated blood pressure.

3. Blood pressure medicines not only lower blood pressure but also contribute to overall heart health by reducing the strain on the heart and blood vessels.

Risks:

1. As with any medication, blood pressure medicines can cause side effects. These may range from mild and temporary to more severe and persistent.

2. In some cases, blood pressure medication may lower blood pressure too much, causing hypotension (abnormally low blood pressure). This may result in dizziness, fainting, or even shock.

3. Combining blood pressure medicines with other medications, supplements, or herbal remedies can sometimes lead to harmful interactions, which may reduce the efficacy of the treatment or cause adverse reactions.

WHAT ARE THE COMMON SIDE EFFECTS OF BLOOD PRESSURE MEDICINES?

The common side effects of blood pressure medicines vary depending on the specific medication and the individual's response to the treatment. Some common side effects include:

1. **Dizziness or lightheadedness:** This may occur when the blood pressure drops too quickly, causing a temporary reduction in blood flow to the brain.
2. **Fatigue:** Some blood pressure medications, particularly beta-blockers, may cause feelings of tiredness or fatigue.
3. **Dry cough**: ACE inhibitors are known to cause a persistent dry cough in some individuals. In these patients, an ARB is a good alternative.
4. **Swelling in the legs, ankles, or feet:** Calcium channel blockers may cause fluid retention, leading to swelling in the lower extremities.
5. **Erectile dysfunction:** Some blood pressure medicines, such as diuretics and beta-blockers, may contribute to erectile dysfunction in men.
6. **Gastrointestinal issues:** Nausea, diarrhea, or constipation may occur as side effects of some blood pressure medications.

7. **Headaches:** Some individuals may experience headaches as a side effect of blood pressure medicines, particularly when starting a new medication or adjusting the dosage.

8. **Insomnia:** Certain blood pressure medications, such as beta-blockers, may cause difficulty falling or staying asleep.

9. **Skin rash:** In some cases, individuals may develop a skin rash or sensitivity to sunlight while taking blood pressure medicines.

10. **Weight gain**: Some blood pressure medications, particularly beta-blockers, may cause weight gain due to fluid retention or changes in metabolism.

It's essential to discuss any side effects you experience with your healthcare provider. In many cases, side effects can be managed or resolved by adjusting the medication dosage or switching to a different medication.

HOW DO YOU KNOW IF YOU NEED MEDICINE FOR HIGH BLOOD PRESSURE?

Determining whether you need medicine for high blood pressure involves several factors, including your blood pressure levels, overall health, and the presence of other risk factors or conditions.

1. Healthcare providers use specific guidelines to determine whether an individual requires medication for high blood pressure. Generally, if your blood pressure consistently measures 140/90 mm Hg or higher, your healthcare provider may consider prescribing medication.

2. If your blood pressure is mildly elevated, your healthcare provider may recommend lifestyle changes, such as a healthy diet, regular exercise, weight loss, stress management, and reducing alcohol and tobacco consumption. If these lifestyle modifications are insufficient in lowering blood pressure, medication may become necessary.

3. If you have other health conditions, such as diabetes, kidney disease, or heart disease, your healthcare provider may prescribe medication to manage your blood pressure more aggressively, even if it's only mildly elevated.

This approach is aimed at reducing the risk of complications associated with high blood pressure.

4. Older individuals may require medication to manage their blood pressure, as the risk of complications increases with age.

5. If you have a family history of high blood pressure or related complications, your healthcare provider may recommend medication as a preventive measure.

It's essential to work closely with your healthcare provider to determine the most appropriate course of action for managing your high blood pressure. Regular blood pressure monitoring, medical checkups, and open communication with your healthcare provider will ensure that you receive the most effective treatment plan tailored to your individual needs.

CLASSES OF BLOOD PRESSURE MEDICATIONS

As we navigate through the world of blood pressure medications, it's essential to understand the various classes of these medicines. Each class has a distinct mechanism of action, which determines how they help control blood pressure. I will guide you through the different classes, discussing their mechanisms and possible side effects and providing examples for each. Let's begin!

1. Diuretics

Diuretics, sometimes known as "water pills," work by helping the kidneys expel excess water and sodium from the body. By reducing fluid volume, these medications decrease the pressure exerted on blood vessels, ultimately lowering blood pressure. There are several types of diuretics which include thiazides, potassium-sparing, loop, and combination. Each category works on a different area within the kidneys. You may be prescribed multiple diuretics from different categories. Many of these medications deplete potassium levels except for potassium-sparing diuretics. It is important to maintain potassium in your diet or supplements to prevent weakness, fatigue, and muscle cramps.

Possible side effects:

- Increased urination
- Dizziness or lightheadedness
- Electrolyte imbalances (such as low potassium levels)
- Dehydration
- Fatigue

- Muscle cramps

Examples:

Thiazide Diuretics

- Chlorthalidone
- Hydrochlorothiazide (Microzide)
- Indapamide
- Metolazone (Zaroxolyn)

Potassium-Sparing Diuretics

- Amiloride
- Spironolactone (Aldactone)
- Triamterene
- Eplerenone (Inspra)

Loop Diuretics

- Furosemide (Lasix)
- Bumetanide (Bumex)

Combination Diuretics

- Amiloride + Hydrochlorothiazide (Moduretic)
- Spironolactone + Hydrochlorothiazide (Aldactazide)
- Triamterene + Hydrochlorothiazide (Maxzide, Dyazide)

2. Beta-blockers

Beta-blockers function by blocking the effects of the hormone epinephrine (adrenaline), which helps slow down the heart rate and reduce the force with which the heart pumps blood. Consequently, this results in decreased blood pressure.

Possible side effects:

- Fatigue or lethargy
- Cold hands and feet
- Dizziness or lightheadedness
- Dry mouth, eyes, or skin
- Insomnia
- Weight gain
- Erectile dysfunction

Examples:

- Atenolol (Tenormin)
- Bisoprolol (Zebeta)
- Metoprolol tartrate (Lopressor)
- Metoprolol succinate (Toprol-XL)
- Propranolol (Inderal)
- Sotalol (Betapace)
- Nadolol (Corgard)
- Acebutolol (Sectral)

Combination Beta-Blocker and Thiazide Diuretic

- Bisoprolol + Hydrochlorothiazide (Ziac)

3. Calcium channel blockers

Calcium channel blockers inhibit the movement of calcium into the muscle cells of the heart and blood vessels. By doing so, these medications relax the blood vessels and reduce the force of the heart's contractions, leading to a decline in blood pressure.

Possible side effects:

- Swelling in the legs, ankles, or feet
- Constipation
- Headaches
- Dizziness or lightheadedness
- Flushing or redness in the face
- Rapid or irregular heartbeat (palpitations)

Examples:

- Amlodipine (Norvasc)
- Diltiazem (Cardizem)
- Felodipine (Plendil)
- Nifedipine (Procardia, Adalat)
- Verapamil (Calan, Verelan)
- Nicardipine (Cardene)

4. ACE inhibitors

Angiotensin-converting enzyme (ACE) inhibitors work by preventing the production of angiotensin II, a hormone that causes blood vessels to constrict. This inhibition results in the relaxation of blood vessels, effectively lowering blood pressure. It is important to note that pregnant women should not take ACE Inhibitors.

Possible side effects:

- Dry, persistent cough
- Dizziness or lightheadedness
- Headaches
- Fatigue
- Swelling in the face or throat (angioedema)
- Elevated potassium levels (hyperkalemia)

Examples:

- Benazepril (Lotensin)
- Captopril (Capoten)
- Enalapril (Vasotec)
- Lisinopril (Prinivil, Zestril)
- Ramipril (Altace)
- Fosinopril (Monopril)
- Quinapril (Accupril)

5. Angiotensin II receptor blockers (ARBs)

Angiotensin II receptor blockers (ARBs) block the action of angiotensin II by preventing it from binding to its receptors. This interference results in relaxed blood vessels and decreased blood pressure, much like ACE inhibitors. It is important to note that pregnant women should not take ARBs.

Possible side effects:

- Dizziness or lightheadedness
- Headaches
- Fatigue
- Elevated potassium levels (hyperkalemia)
- Swelling in the face or throat (angioedema)— although this is less common than with ACE inhibitors.

Examples:

- Losartan (Cozaar)
- Valsartan (Diovan)
- Irbesartan (Avapro)
- Candesartan (Atacand)
- Olmesartan (Benicar)
- Telmisartan (Micardis)

6. Alpha-blockers

Alpha-blockers work by blocking alpha receptors on the smooth muscles of blood vessels, which leads to the relaxation of these muscles. This reduces resistance in the blood vessels and lowers blood pressure.

Possible side effects:

- Dizziness or lightheadedness, primarily upon standing (orthostatic hypotension)
- Rapid or irregular heartbeat (palpitations)
- Headaches
- Fatigue
- Fluid retention, leading to swelling in the legs, ankles, or feet

Examples:

- Prazosin (Minipress)
- Terazosin (Hytrin)
- Doxazosin (Cardura)

7. Alpha-beta-blockers

Alpha-beta blockers combine the actions of alpha-blockers and beta-blockers. They block both alpha receptors and beta receptors, relaxing blood vessels and slowing down the heart rate. This dual action results in lowered blood pressure.

Possible side effects:

- Dizziness or lightheadedness, primarily upon standing (orthostatic hypotension)

- Fatigue
- Headaches
- Cold hands and feet
- Rapid or irregular heartbeat (palpitations)
- Erectile dysfunction

Examples:

- Carvedilol (Coreg)
- Labetalol (Trandate, Normodyne)

8. Central-acting agents

Central-acting agents work on the brain, reducing the signals sent to the nervous system that constrict blood vessels and increase heart rate. By decreasing these signals, these medications help lower blood pressure.

Possible side effects:

- Dizziness or lightheadedness
- Dry mouth
- Constipation
- Fatigue or drowsiness
- Erectile dysfunction

Examples:

- Clonidine (Catapres)
- Methyldopa (Aldomet)
- Guanfacine (Tenex)

9. Vasodilators

Vasodilators directly act on the smooth muscles of blood vessels, causing them to relax and widen. This dilation of blood vessels reduces resistance and lowers blood pressure.

Possible side effects:

- Headaches
- Rapid or irregular heartbeat (palpitations)
- Flushing or redness in the face
- Swelling in the legs, ankles, or feet
- Chest pain or discomfort

Examples:

- Hydralazine (Apresoline)
- Minoxidil (Loniten)

10. Aldosterone receptor antagonists

Aldosterone receptor antagonists (ARAs) are a class of medications that inhibit the action of aldosterone, a hormone that regulates salt and water balance in the body. By blocking aldosterone, ARAs promote the excretion of sodium and water and the retention of potassium, helping to reduce blood volume and lower blood pressure. This makes them valuable for managing conditions such as hypertension and heart failure. These are both part of the afore-mentioned potassium-sparing diuretics.

Possible side effects:

- Hyperkalemia (increased potassium levels in the blood)
- Gynecomastia (breast enlargement in males)
- Menstrual irregularities
- Impotence
- Kidney function abnormalities

Examples:

- Spironolactone (Aldactone)
- Eplerenone (Inspra)

11. Direct renin inhibitors

Direct renin inhibitors (DRIs) are a type of medication that works to control hypertension by directly inhibiting renin, an enzyme that triggers a sequence of reactions leading to blood vessel constriction and sodium retention. By blocking renin, these drugs help relax blood vessels and reduce fluid retention, effectively lowering blood pressure.

Possible side effects:

- Dizziness or lightheadedness
- Cough
- Diarrhea
- Flu-like symptoms
- Fatigue
- Elevated potassium levels in the blood (hyperkalemia)

Examples:

- Aliskiren (Tekturna or Rasilez)

As we've explored the different classes of blood pressure medications, it's essential to remember that each person's needs are unique. A healthcare provider can help you determine the best medication or combination of medications for your situation.

It's also crucial to communicate any side effects you experience with your healthcare provider, as they may need to adjust your treatment plan accordingly. Together, you can work toward effectively managing your high blood pressure and maintaining optimal health.

COMBINATION THERAPY

Managing high blood pressure often requires a comprehensive strategy that combines lifestyle modifications and medications. Addressing your diet, exercise, stress levels, and smoking habits can significantly impact your blood pressure and help minimize the risk of complications associated with this condition.

However, there are instances where lifestyle adjustments alone may not suffice to bring your blood pressure down to a healthy range. In such cases, medication may be necessary to assist in lowering your blood pressure.

Your healthcare provider plays a crucial role in recommending the most suitable medication or combination of medications for you. They will take into account your medical history, risk factors, and overall health status.

When it comes to treating high blood pressure, employing a combination of two or more drugs can improve both blood pressure control and tolerance to the medications. Utilizing two medications with different mechanisms of action can be more effective in lowering blood pressure compared to merely increasing the dose of a single drug.

This approach also enables the use of lower doses for each medication, which can result in fewer side effects and promote adherence to the prescribed treatment. Research has demonstrated that combination therapy can be more effective than relying on a single drug alone, helping individuals with high blood pressure to better manage their condition.

While combination therapy for high blood pressure can yield remarkable results, it is vital to collaborate closely with your healthcare provider to determine the most appropriate combination of medications tailored to your needs. It's important to note that not all medications can be safely combined, and certain combinations may lead to interactions or side effects that could be detrimental to your health.

To better understand the benefits of combination therapy, let's explore some of the reasons why it can be a more practical approach:

1. Enhanced blood pressure control

By targeting different aspects of the blood pressure regulation system, combination therapy can provide a more comprehensive approach to managing high blood pressure. For example, combining a diuretic, which removes excess fluid from the body, with a beta-blocker, which reduces the heart rate and force of contraction, can result in more effective blood pressure control than using either drug alone.

2. Minimized side effects

Since combination therapy often involves lower doses of each medication, the risk of side effects can be reduced. Lower doses also make it easier for patients to tolerate the medications, increasing the likelihood of adherence to the treatment plan.

3. Improved treatment adherence

Taking multiple medications can be challenging for some individuals, but combination therapy can simplify the process. Many pharmaceutical companies offer fixed-dose combination pills, which contain two or more blood pressure-lowering medications in a single tablet. This can make it more convenient for patients to take their medications as prescribed, improving treatment adherence and overall blood pressure control.

4. Faster blood pressure reduction

In some cases, using combination therapy can lead to a quicker reduction in blood pressure. This can be particularly beneficial for individuals with severely elevated blood pressure or those at high risk for complications related to high blood pressure.

Despite its benefits, it's essential to recognize that combination therapy is not without potential drawbacks. Some of the challenges associated with this approach include:

1. Drug interactions

Combining multiple medications increases the risk of drug interactions, which can either reduce the effectiveness of the medications or cause harmful side effects. It's crucial to discuss all medications you're taking, including over-the-counter drugs and supplements, with your healthcare provider to minimize this risk.

2. Increased cost

Using multiple medications can lead to higher treatment costs, which may be a barrier for some individuals. However, the potential for improved blood pressure control and reduced risk of complications may offset these costs in the long run.

3. Complexity of treatment

Managing multiple medications can be complex, particularly for older adults or those with cognitive impairments. It's essential to work closely with your healthcare provider and develop strategies to simplify your treatment regimen and ensure proper medication management and adherence.

To overcome these challenges, and maximize the benefits of combination therapy, consider the following strategies:

1. Open communication with your healthcare provider

Maintain an open dialogue with your healthcare provider about your symptoms, concerns, and the medications you're taking. This will enable them to better understand your unique needs and monitor your progress while adjusting your treatment plan as needed.

2. Adherence to your treatment plan

Following your prescribed treatment plan is crucial for achieving optimal blood pressure control. Remember to take your medications as directed and notify your healthcare provider if you experience any side effects or challenges with adherence.

3. Regular monitoring of blood pressure

Regularly monitoring your blood pressure, either at home or through visits to your healthcare provider, will help you and your provider assess the effectiveness of your treatment plan and make necessary adjustments. Home blood pressure monitoring can be especially helpful in identifying the impact of lifestyle modifications and medication changes on your blood pressure.

4. Lifestyle modifications

In addition to combination therapy, continue to prioritize lifestyle changes, such as healthy eating, regular exercise, stress management, and smoking cessation. These modifications can not only help lower your blood pressure but also improve your overall health and well-being.

5. Stay informed and proactive

Educate yourself about high blood pressure and the various medications used to treat it. Being informed and proactive about your health can help you make more informed decisions and engage in meaningful discussions with your healthcare provider.

In essence, combination therapy can be a highly effective approach for managing high blood pressure, particularly when paired with lifestyle modifications. By working closely with your healthcare provider, carefully monitoring your blood pressure, and adhering to your treatment plan, you can take control of your high blood pressure and work toward a healthier future.

Remember, each person's journey with high blood pressure is unique, and finding the right combination of medications and lifestyle changes may take time, but with persistence and support from your healthcare team, you can achieve better blood pressure control and improve your overall quality of life.

HYPERTENSION MEDICATION INTERACTION WITH OTC DRUGS

Hypertensive medications play a critical role in managing high blood pressure, but they can also interact with various foods, supplements, and over-the-counter (OTC) drugs. These interactions can influence the effectiveness of your blood pressure medications or heighten the risk of side effects. It's crucial to exercise caution when taking hypertension medications and to consult your healthcare provider about any potential interactions.

Your healthcare provider may suggest avoiding specific foods, supplements, or OTC drugs or modify the dosage of your medication to prevent undesired inter-actions. Here are some key points to consider when using hypertension medications in conjunction with OTC drugs:

1. Over-the-counter pain relievers

Nonsteroidal anti-inflammatory drugs (NSAIDs) like ibuprofen, aspirin, and naproxen are commonly used OTC pain relievers. However, these medications can reduce the effectiveness of certain blood pressure medications and even cause your blood pressure to rise. If you require a pain reliever, it's advisable to discuss the safest options with your healthcare provider, who may recommend alternatives like acetaminophen.

2. Cold and flu medications

Decongestants such as phenylephrine and pseudoephedrine are found in many cold and flu medications which can elevate your blood pressure and interfere with the effectiveness of your hypertension medications. Before taking any cold or flu remedies, consult your healthcare provider or pharmacist to ensure they are safe for you to use.

3. Herbal supplements

Some herbal supplements, such as St. John's Wort, ginkgo biloba, and ginseng, can interact with blood pressure medications, altering their effectiveness or increasing the risk of side effects. Before starting any herbal supplement, discuss your intentions with your healthcare provider, who can advise you on potential interactions and safety concerns.

4. Antacids and acid reducers

Some antacids and acid reducers, like calcium carbonate or proton pump inhibitors, can interfere with the absorption of certain blood pressure medications. If you need to take these medications, consult your healthcare provider about possible interactions and the best time to take them to minimize any adverse effects.

5. Caffeine

While it is not an OTC medication, it's essential to be mindful of your caffeine intake when taking hypertension medications. Caffeine can cause a temporary spike in blood pressure, which could counteract the effects of your medications. Monitor your caffeine consumption and discuss any concerns with your healthcare provider.

6. Alcohol

Similar to caffeine, alcohol can impact your blood pressure and interact with your hypertension medications. Excessive alcohol consumption can raise your blood pressure and reduce the effectiveness of your medications. It's crucial to limit alcohol intake and follow your healthcare provider's recommendations.

To sum it up, it's vital to be cautious and well-informed when using hypertension medications in combination with OTC drugs, supplements, or certain substances like caffeine and alcohol. Regular communication with your healthcare provider can help you navigate potential interactions, ensuring your medications are working effectively and safely.

COMMON HIGH BLOOD PRESSURE MEDICATION INTERACTIONS

High blood pressure medication interactions can occur with various substances, including food, beverages, dietary supplements, and other drugs. Understanding these interactions is essential for the safe and effective management of high blood pressure. Let's delve into some common interactions that you should be aware of:

Drugs with Food and Beverages

Certain foods and beverages can interact with high blood pressure medications, impacting their effectiveness or causing side effects. For instance:

- Grapefruit juice: This beverage can interfere with the metabolism of some calcium channel blockers, causing an increase in drug levels and potentially leading to side effects.

- Potassium-rich foods: Consuming large amounts of potassium-rich foods while taking potassium-sparing diuretics can lead to dangerously high potassium levels in the blood, which can cause heart rhythm problems.
- Alcohol: Excessive alcohol consumption can raise blood pressure and reduce the effectiveness of high blood pressure medications.

It's essential to discuss any dietary concerns with your healthcare provider to minimize potential interactions and maintain the effectiveness of your medications.

Drugs with Dietary Supplements

Dietary supplements can also interact with high blood pressure medications:

- Coenzyme Q10 (CoQ10): While CoQ10 is often used for heart health, it can interfere with the effectiveness of certain blood pressure medications, like beta-blockers and diuretics.
- St. John's Wort: This herbal supplement may interact with blood pressure medications, altering their effectiveness or increasing the risk of side effects.

- Potassium supplements: Similar to potassium-rich foods, potassium supplements can be problematic when taken with potassium-sparing diuretics, leading to dangerously high potassium levels.

Before starting any dietary supplement, consult your healthcare provider to avoid potential interactions.

Drugs with Other Drugs

High blood pressure medications can also interact with other prescription and over-the-counter drugs, including:

- **Antihistamines**: These medications, commonly used to treat allergy symptoms, can counteract the blood pressure-lowering effects of certain medications, like alpha-blockers.
- **Bronchodilators:** Asthma medications, such as albuterol, can cause an increase in heart rate and blood pressure. This may interfere with the effectiveness of your high blood pressure medications.
- **Cordarone (amiodarone):** This antiarrhythmic drug can interact with beta-blockers and calcium channel blockers,

potentially causing dangerous heart rhythm disturbances.

- **Nasal decongestants**: Decongestants found in cold and allergy medications can raise blood pressure and interfere with the effectiveness of high blood pressure medications.
- **Nicotine replacement products:** Nicotine, whether from smoking or replacement products, can raise blood pressure and counteract the effects of high blood pressure medications.

To avoid harmful drug interactions, inform your healthcare provider of all medications and supplements you are taking.

In summary, it's crucial to be aware of common high blood pressure medication interactions with food, beverages, dietary supplements, and other drugs. These interactions can impact the effectiveness of your medications or increase the risk of side effects.

By discussing potential interactions with your health-care provider and following their guidance, you can safely manage your high blood pressure and avoid complications. Stay informed, be proactive, and maintain open communication with your healthcare team to ensure the best possible outcomes in your high blood pressure management journey.

TIPS TO AVOID INTERACTIONS

To avoid interactions between high blood pressure medications and other substances, it's essential to take proactive steps and maintain open communication with your healthcare team. Here are some practical tips to help minimize potential interactions and ensure the safe and effective management of your high blood pressure:

1. Ensure all your healthcare providers are aware of all the medicines you are taking, including prescription drugs, over-the-counter medications, dietary and herbal supplements, and vitamins. This will enable them to better evaluate any potential interactions and recommend suitable treatments.

2. Before taking any new medication, consult your healthcare provider or pharmacist and ask essential questions, such as whether the new drug will interact with your current medications, the best time to take it, and possible side effects.

3. Drug interaction checkers, available online or as mobile apps, can help you identify potential interactions between your medications. While these tools can be helpful, they should not replace professional advice from your healthcare provider.

4. Carefully read the labels of all over-the-counter and prescription medications you take. Labels often contain crucial information about potential interactions and side effects.

5. By using one pharmacy for all your prescriptions, you can ensure that the pharmacist has a complete record of your medications, making it easier for them to identify potential interactions and provide personalized guidance.

Remember, managing high blood pressure is an ongoing process, and it's crucial to stay informed, proactive, and engaged in your treatment plan. With the support of your healthcare team and the adoption of these practical tips, you can achieve better blood pressure control and enjoy a healthier future.

QUESTIONS TO ASK YOUR HEALTHCARE PROVIDER

Before starting any medication for high blood pressure, it's essential to have an open and thorough conversation with your healthcare provider to ensure the chosen medication is both safe and effective for your specific needs. To help guide your discussion, here are ten important questions you should consider asking your doctor or pharmacist:

1. What is the primary function of this medication?

Ask your healthcare provider about the intended purpose of the medication, how it works, and the expected benefits for your blood pressure management.

2. How and when should I take this medication?

Inquire about the appropriate dosage, timing, and whether the medication should be taken with or without food. This information is crucial to ensure proper absorption and effectiveness.

3. Can I take this medication with other drugs?

Discuss potential interactions with other medications you are currently taking and learn about any warning signs of adverse drug interactions.

4. Are there possible side effects or interactions with food or supplements?

Understand the potential side effects and any interactions with specific foods, beverages, or dietary supplements that could affect the medication's effectiveness or safety.

5. How long will it take before the medication begins to work?

Ask your healthcare provider about the expected time frame for the medication to start showing its effects on your blood pressure.

6. How can I determine if the medication is working, and how frequently should I monitor my blood pressure?

Learn how to evaluate the effectiveness of your

medication and the recommended frequency for blood pressure monitoring.

7. Are there any lifestyle changes I should make while taking this medication?

Discuss any recommended adjustments to your diet, exercise routine, or other lifestyle factors that may complement your high blood pressure treatment plan.

8. What precautions should I take while on this medication?

Understand any specific precautions you should be aware of while taking the medication, such as avoiding particular activities, foods, or beverages.

9. What should I do if I miss a dose or accidentally take too much medication?

Learn the appropriate steps to take in case you miss a dose or accidentally take more medication than prescribed.

10. When should I schedule a follow-up appointment to assess my blood pressure and evaluate the medication's effectiveness?

Determine the optimal time for a follow-up appointment to review your blood pressure levels and discuss the medication's effectiveness with your healthcare provider.

By asking these vital questions and staying informed about your medication and its potential interactions, you can better manage your high blood pressure and reduce the risk of complications. Remember, active involvement in your treatment plan and open communication with your healthcare team is key to achieving optimal blood pressure control and improving your overall health.

As we wrap up this chapter, I hope I've been able to provide you with a solid understanding of the different medications available for managing high blood pressure and the crucial steps to avoid harmful drug interactions. Remember, knowledge and communication are key to ensuring the safe and effective use of these medications.

In the upcoming chapter, we'll dive into the world of dietary modifications and explore various ways to effectively and safely lower your blood pressure through changes in your eating habits. This valuable information can make a significant difference in your blood pressure management journey.

4

HEALTHY FOOD FOR A HAPPY HEART

A s we unveil the secrets to a rejuvenated life in this chapter, you'll discover transformative diet modifications to safely reduce blood pressure and enhance overall well-being. In Jim Rohn's words: *"Take care of your body. It's the only place you have to live."* After all, keeping yourself well informed about your health and actively pursuing lifestyle adjustment knowledge is imperative.

Another measure to enhance your well-being is to ultimately become your own strongest supporter. Minor changes to your everyday habits, like incorporating consistent physical activity, embracing a nutritious diet, and regulating stress levels, can decrease your blood pressure and diminish the risks linked to hypertension.

YOUR DIET AND HEART HEALTH: A CRUCIAL CONNECTION

The food choices we make significantly impact our heart health. By embracing diets that promote cardiovascular well-being, we can lower the risk of heart disease. One such diet is the DASH (Dietary Approaches to Stop Hypertension) diet.

THE DASH DIET: A LIFELINE FOR YOUR HEART

The DASH diet is nutrient-rich and designed to lower blood pressure and protect your heart. Focusing on consuming whole foods encourages a balanced intake of fruits, vegetables, whole grains, lean proteins, and low-fat dairy products.

Potential Benefits of the DASH Diet

Adopting the DASH diet may reduce blood pressure, improve cholesterol levels, and decrease the risk of heart disease and stroke. It can also promote weight loss and support overall health.

DASH Diet Suitability

While the DASH diet is generally beneficial, individual results may vary. Consulting a healthcare professional is recommended to determine if it's the right fit for your unique health needs.

Salt Restriction: Striking the Right Balance

Excess salt consumption can contribute to high blood pressure, but overly restricting salt may negatively affect the body's sodium balance. Finding a moderate approach is essential, following recommended daily intake guidelines.

DASH Diet Foods: Dos and Don'ts

Enjoy Fruits, vegetables, whole grains, lean meats, fish, poultry, nuts, seeds, legumes, and low-fat dairy products. Avoid Processed foods, high-sodium items, saturated fats, sugary beverages, and excessive alcohol.

Sample Menu

A well-planned DASH diet menu incorporates a variety of whole foods, providing diverse flavors and nutrients. A sample week might include whole-grain oatmeal with berries, grilled chicken salads, brown rice with steamed vegetables, and baked fish with quinoa.

▷ *Day 1: Menu*

Breakfast

- 1 cup of oatmeal without salt
- 1/4 cup raisins
- 1 medium banana
- 1 cup fat-free milk
- Coffee, tea, or water

Lunch

- Hummus plate with:

  - 1/2 cup hummus
  - 1/2 medium red pepper
  - 1/2 medium cucumber
  - 10 baby carrots
  - 1 whole-grain pita pocket

- Water

Dinner

- Roasted salmon with:

  ○ 4 ounces of salmon
  ○ Maple balsamic glaze

- 1 cup whole-grain and wild rice blend
- 3/4 cup green beans with red bell peppers
- 1/2 cup canned pear slices in juice
- Tea, hot or cold, and not sweetened

Snack (anytime)

- 1 cup low-fat yogurt
- 1 medium peach

▷ *Day 2: Menu*

Breakfast

- 1 cup mixed fruit such as melon and grapes
- 1/2 whole-wheat bagel
- 1 tablespoon natural peanut butter
- 1 cup skim milk
- Coffee, tea, or water.

Lunch

- Spinach salad with:

  - 3 cups fresh spinach leaves
  - 1 sliced pear
  - 1/2 cup canned mandarin oranges
  - 1 tablespoon red wine vinegar
  - 1 tablespoon olive oil
  - 1 ounce of goat cheese
  - 3 ounces of cooked chicken

- 1 small whole-wheat roll
- Water

Dinner

- Vegetarian pasta with:

  - 1/2 cup marinara sauce
  - 1 cup chopped summer squash
  - 1/2 cup frozen chopped spinach
  - 1 1/2 cups whole-wheat pasta

- 1 cup melon
- 1 cup skim milk

Snack (anytime)

- 1/4 cup trail mix, not salted

▷ *Day 3: Menu*

Breakfast

- 1 whole-grain English muffin
- 1 poached egg
- 1 medium orange
- 1 cup low-fat yogurt
- Herbal tea or water

Lunch

- Quinoa salad with:

  ○ 1 cup cooked quinoa
  ○ Cherry tomatoes
  ○ Cucumber slices
  ○ 1/4 cup feta cheese
  ○ 2 tablespoons balsamic vinaigrette dressing

- Grilled chicken breast (4 ounces)
- 1 medium apple
- Water with lemon

Dinner

- Baked salmon with:

  o Lemon and dill
  o 1 cup steamed broccoli
  o 1/2 cup brown rice

- Mixed berry salad (blueberries, strawberries, raspberries)
- 1 cup skim milk

Snack (anytime)

- 1 small banana
- Handful of raw almonds

Adjusting Your Diet to DASH Guidelines

Follow DASH guidelines, prioritize whole foods, control portion sizes, and minimize processed items. Gradually increase your intake of fruits, vegetables, and whole grains, while reducing saturated fats, sodium, and added sugars. Remember, small changes can make a significant impact on your heart health.

Embracing the DASH Lifestyle: Tips and Strategies

1. **Gradual Change:** Instead of overhauling your diet overnight, make incremental adjustments to ensure a smoother, sustainable transition. This approach can help you adapt to the DASH diet without feeling overwhelmed.

2. **Meal Planning:** Create weekly meal plans to streamline grocery shopping and avoid impulsive, unhealthy food choices. This strategy can save time, reduce stress, and ensure you stay on track with your DASH diet goals.

3. **Mindful Eating:** Pay attention to hunger and satiety cues and savor each bite. By eating slowly and deliberately, you can improve digestion, enjoy your food more, and prevent overeating.

4. **Home Cooking:** Prepare meals at home to control the ingredients and cooking methods, ensuring that your dishes align with DASH guidelines. Experiment with new recipes, flavors, and techniques to keep your meals exciting and satisfying.

5. **Hydration:** Drinking water is essential for overall health and can help with weight management. Stay hydrated by consuming water throughout the day, replacing sugary

beverages with healthier alternatives like herbal tea or infused water.

6. **Support System**: Engage with friends or family members who share your health goals or join online communities centered around the DASH diet. A strong support network can provide encouragement, motivation, and accountability.

7. **Regular Check-Ins**: Monitor your progress by checking blood pressure, weight, and other health indicators. This practice will help you evaluate the effectiveness of the DASH diet and make any necessary adjustments.

Remember, the journey to a healthier heart begins with a single step. Embrace the DASH diet and its principles, and you'll be well on your way to improved cardiovascular health and overall well-being.

THE MEDITERRANEAN DIET: A JOURNEY TO WHOLESOME WELLNESS

The Mediterranean diet is a heart-healthy eating plan inspired by the traditional cuisine of countries bordering the Mediterranean Sea. It emphasizes plant-based foods, healthy fats, and moderate protein consumption, focusing on quality, variety, and balance.

Potential Benefits of the Mediterranean Diet

Adopting this diet may improve cardiovascular health, weight loss, better blood sugar control, and reduce risk of chronic diseases. Its nutrient-dense, antioxidant-rich nature also supports overall well-being and longevity.

Embarking on the Mediterranean Path

To start, gradually incorporate the dietary principles and food choices typical of the Mediterranean lifestyle. Choose whole, minimally processed foods, and explore new flavors and cooking techniques inspired by Mediterranean cuisine.

Foods to Savor

Enjoy a diverse range of plant-based foods like fruits, vegetables, whole grains, nuts, seeds, and legumes. Choose healthy fats such as olive oil, avocados, and fatty fish like salmon and sardines. Consume moderate amounts of lean proteins, including poultry, eggs, and dairy products.

Foods to Limit

Minimize the intake of red meat, processed foods, refined sugars, and unhealthy fats like trans fats and saturated fats. Consume alcohol, particularly red wine, in moderation.

Sample Weekly Menu

A well-crafted Mediterranean diet menu is rich in flavors, colors, and textures. A sample week might include whole-grain salads with fresh vegetables and herbs, grilled fish drizzled with olive oil, lentil soup, vegetable-stuffed peppers, and fresh fruit with yogurt for dessert. Embrace the Mediterranean diet to nourish your body with wholesome, delicious meals, and embark on a journey to enhanced health, vitality, and longevity.

▷ **Monday**

- Breakfast: Greek yogurt with strawberries and chia seeds
- Lunch: A whole-grain sandwich with hummus and vegetables
- Dinner: A tuna salad with greens and olive oil, as well as a fruit salad

▷ Tuesday

- Breakfast: Oatmeal with blueberries
- Lunch: Caprese zucchini noodles with mozzarella, cherry tomatoes, olive oil, and balsamic vinegar
- Dinner: A salad with tomatoes, olives, cucumbers, farro, baked trout, and feta cheese

▷ Wednesday

- Breakfast: An omelet with mushrooms, tomatoes, and onions
- Lunch: A whole-grain sandwich with cheese and fresh vegetables
- Dinner: Mediterranean lasagna

▷ Thursday

- Breakfast: Yogurt with sliced fruit and nuts
- Lunch: A quinoa salad with chickpeas
- Dinner: Broiled salmon with brown rice and vegetables

▷ **Friday**

- Breakfast: Eggs and sautéed vegetables with whole-wheat toast
- Lunch: Stuffed zucchini boats with pesto, turkey sausage, tomatoes, bell peppers, and cheese
- Dinner: Grilled lamb with salad and baked potato

▷ **Saturday**

- Breakfast: Oatmeal with nuts and raisins or apple slices
- Lunch: Lentil salad with feta, tomatoes, cucumbers, and olives
- Dinner: Mediterranean pizza made with whole-wheat pita bread and topped with cheese, vegetables, and olives

▷ **Sunday**

- Breakfast: An omelet with veggies and olives
- Lunch: Bowl with feta, onions, tomatoes, hummus, and rice
- Dinner: Grilled chicken with vegetables, sweet potato fries, and fresh fruit

There's usually no need to count calories or track macronutrients (protein, fat, and carbs) on the Mediterranean diet unless you are managing your glucose levels. It is essential to consume all foods in moderation and not overindulge.

DIETARY WISDOM FOR A HEALTHY HEART: PRACTICAL TIPS AND TRICKS

Caring for your heart is paramount, and the choices you make at the dining table play a crucial role in safeguarding your cardiovascular well-being. Here are some essential diet tips to help you maintain a healthy heart:

1. Portion Control: Master the Art

Overeating can lead to weight gain, increasing the risk of heart disease. Learning to control portion sizes is key to maintaining a healthy weight and reducing cardiovascular strain. Use smaller plates, check serving sizes on food labels, and listen to your body's hunger and satiety cues to avoid overindulging.

2. A Colorful Plate: Embrace Vegetables and Fruits

Vegetables and fruits are abundant in vitamins, minerals, fiber, and antioxidants that support heart health. Aim to fill half of your plate with a colorful variety of these nutrient powerhouses. Incorporate them into your meals as salads, side dishes, or even as healthy snacks between meals.

3. The Wholesome Choice: Choose Whole Grains

Whole grains, such as brown rice, quinoa, oats, and whole wheat, are rich in fiber and essential nutrients that help regulate blood pressure and cholesterol levels. Replace refined grains with whole-grain options to enhance heart health and maintain steady blood sugar levels.

4. Fats: Discerning the Good from the Bad

Not all fats are created equal. Prioritize heart-healthy fats, like those found in olive oil, nuts, seeds, and avocados, while limiting unhealthy fats, such as trans fats and saturated fats found in processed and fried foods. Moderation is key, even with healthy fats, as they are calorie-dense.

5. Protein Power: Lean and Low-Fat

Choose low-fat protein sources, such as lean meats, poultry, fish, beans, legumes, and low-fat dairy products. Fish, particularly fatty varieties like salmon and mackerel, are rich in omega-3 fatty acids that promote heart health. Aim to incorporate at least two servings of fish per week.

6. Sodium Savvy: Tread Lightly on Salt

Excessive sodium intake can elevate blood pressure, increasing the risk of heart disease. Limit processed foods, which are often high in salt, and season your meals with herbs, spices, and other low-sodium flavor enhancers. Aim to stay within the recommended daily sodium intake guidelines.

7. Planning for Success: Crafting Daily Menus

Planning your meals in advance enables you to make healthier choices and avoid impulsive, less nutritious options. Create a balanced menu that incorporates heart-healthy foods and allows for some flexibility. A well-planned menu helps you stay on track with your dietary goals and streamlines meal preparation.

8. Indulge Mindfully: The Joy of Occasional Treats

A heart-healthy diet doesn't mean completely depriving yourself of the foods you love. Allowing yourself an occasional treat can prevent feelings of deprivation and help you stay committed to your healthy eating habits. Enjoy these indulgences mindfully and in moderation.

By incorporating these practical tips into your daily life, you can cultivate a heart-healthy diet that not only supports your cardiovascular system but also enhances your overall well-being. Remember, every small change adds up to make a significant impact on your health.

What about caffeine?

Caffeine, a naturally occurring stimulant found in coffee, has become an integral part of many people's daily routines. However, its effects on blood pressure have raised concerns, especially for individuals with hypertension. Let's delve into the connection between caffeine and blood pressure.

1. Coffee's Pressure Push: The Mechanics

Caffeine can cause a temporary increase in blood pressure by stimulating the release of stress hormones, such as adrenaline, which in turn constrict blood vessels and raise the heart rate. The exact duration and magnitude of this effect may vary based on individual factors like genetics, tolerance, and caffeine sensitivity.

2. The Long Haul: Prolonged Coffee Consumption

While the short-term effects of caffeine on blood pressure are well established, the long-term impact is less clear. Some studies suggest that regular coffee consumption may be associated with a slightly increased risk of developing hypertension, while others indicate that the body can develop a tolerance to these effects over time. More research is needed to fully understand the long-term implications of habitual coffee drinking.

3. Hypertension and Coffee: Navigating the Dilemma

For those with hypertension, it is crucial to monitor and manage blood pressure. While there is no one-size-fits-all answer, individuals with high blood pressure should consider their unique circumstances when deciding on coffee consumption.

Some may be more sensitive to caffeine's effects and should limit their intake, while others might experience little to no impact on their blood pressure. Consulting with a healthcare professional is recommended to determine the best course of action.

4. Decaf Dynamics: A Milder Jolt

Decaffeinated coffee contains only a fraction of the caffeine found in regular coffee, making it a viable alternative for those looking to minimize caffeine's effects on blood pressure. However, even decaf coffee may still cause a slight, short-lived increase in blood pressure for some individuals. Paying attention to your body's response is essential in determining whether decaf coffee is a suitable option.

5. Time to Pause: Ceasing Coffee Consumption

If you find that coffee consumption significantly raises your blood pressure or exacerbates hypertension, it may be time to consider reducing or stopping your intake. Gradually decreasing your coffee consumption can help prevent withdrawal symptoms such as headaches, fatigue, and irritability.

6. Beyond the Bean: Coffee Alternatives

For those looking to reduce or eliminate coffee consumption, several alternatives can provide a comforting ritual without blood pressure concerns. Herbal teas, like chamomile or peppermint, offer warmth and flavor without caffeine.

Green tea, while still containing some caffeine, has a lower amount than coffee and provides antioxidants that promote health. Chicory root coffee, a caffeine-free option, mimics the taste and aroma of coffee and can be a satisfying substitute.

Understanding the relationship between caffeine and blood pressure is essential for making informed decisions about your coffee consumption. Listen to your body, consult with a healthcare professional, and explore alternatives to find the right balance for your health and well-being.

7. Caffeine in Perspective: A Holistic Approach

When assessing the effects of caffeine on blood pressure, it's important to consider the broader context of your lifestyle and overall health. Factors such as diet, exercise, stress management, and sleep quality all play a significant role in determining your blood pressure and heart health.

8. Mindful Consumption: Know Your Limits

Being aware of your personal caffeine tolerance and sensitivity can help you make more informed choices about coffee consumption. Pay attention to how your body reacts to caffeine and adjust your intake accordingly. It is generally recommended not to exceed 400 mg of caffeine per day, which is roughly equivalent to four 8-ounce cups of brewed coffee.

9. Caffeine and Beyond Coffee's Nutrient Profile

While the focus is often on caffeine's impact on blood pressure, it's essential to recognize that coffee also contains various beneficial compounds, including antioxidants and polyphenols. These bioactive compounds can help reduce inflammation, protect against cellular damage, and support overall health. Moderation is key—enjoy the potential benefits without overdoing it.

10. Caffeine and Lifestyle: Striking a Balance

When looking to manage blood pressure and maintain heart health, a comprehensive approach that encompasses various aspects of your lifestyle is crucial. In addition to monitoring your caffeine intake, focus on eating a balanced diet rich in whole foods, engaging in regular physical activity, managing stress through techniques like meditation or yoga, and getting adequate, restful sleep.

Navigating the complex relationship between caffeine and blood pressure requires self-awareness, knowledge, and adaptability. By incorporating a holistic approach to your health and considering your unique circumstances, you can make well-informed decisions about coffee consumption that support your overall well-being and heart health. Embrace a balanced lifestyle and enjoy your coffee—or alternatives—mindfully and responsibly.

HEART-HEALTHY PANTRY: 21 FOODS TO NOURISH AND PROTECT YOUR HEART

1. **Fresh Herbs:** Flavorful alternatives to salt, these aromatic plants help reduce sodium intake and support heart health.
2. **Black Beans:** Rich in fiber and protein, these legumes lower cholesterol and maintain stable blood sugar levels.
3. **Red Wine and Resveratrol:** Moderate consumption of red wine, containing the

antioxidant resveratrol, may protect against heart disease.

4. **Salmon:** This superfood is packed with omega-3 fatty acids, which decrease inflammation and improve cardiovascular function.

5. **Tuna:** Another excellent source of omega-3s, tuna supports heart health and reduces inflammation.

6. **Olive Oil:** Rich in heart-healthy monounsaturated fats, olive oil can help lower bad cholesterol and reduce the risk of heart disease.

7. **Walnuts:** These nuts provide essential nutrients, including omega-3s, antioxidants, and fiber, promoting a healthy heart.

8. **Almonds:** High in monounsaturated fats, almonds help lower cholesterol levels and improve heart health.

9. **Edamame:** Soybeans are a great source of plant-based protein, fiber, and heart-healthy nutrients.

10. **Tofu:** Another soy-based option, tofu is low in saturated fat and high in nutrients, supporting heart health.

11. **Sweet Potatoes:** Packed with vitamins, minerals, and fiber, these tubers help regulate blood pressure and maintain heart health.

12. **Oranges:** Rich in potassium and vitamin C, oranges support healthy blood pressure and protect the cardiovascular system.
13. **Swiss Chard:** This leafy green is high in magnesium and potassium, essential minerals for heart health.
14. **Barley:** A whole grain containing soluble fiber, barley helps lower cholesterol and supports cardiovascular well-being.
15. **Oatmeal:** Rich in fiber and nutrients, oatmeal reduces cholesterol levels and improves heart health.
16. **Flaxseed:** A plant-based source of omega-3 fatty acids, flaxseed promotes heart health and reduces inflammation.
17. **Low-Fat Yogurt:** A probiotic-rich source of calcium and protein, low-fat yogurt supports a healthy heart.
18. **Foods Fortified with Sterols:** These plant compounds help lower cholesterol levels, promoting heart health.
19. **Cherries:** With anti-inflammatory and antioxidant properties, cherries help protect the heart.
20. **Blueberries:** Packed with antioxidants, these berries support heart health and reduce inflammation.

21. **Dark Leafy Greens:** Nutrient-dense and rich in antioxidants, leafy greens like spinach and kale contribute to a healthy heart.

Incorporate these 21 heart-healthy foods into your diet to nourish and protect your cardiovascular system, promoting overall well-being. Altering your dietary habits can significantly contribute to reducing your blood pressure.

However, it is essential to remember that a comprehensive approach to managing high blood pressure also involves exercise and weight management. In the next chapter, we will explore the vital roles that physical activity and sustaining a healthy weight play in safely and effectively lowering your blood pressure. By doing so, you can decrease your chances of developing heart disease and enhance your general well-being. It's time to embrace an active lifestyle and embark on the journey toward optimal health!

5

MOVE IT AND LOSE IT

> "*Even when all is known, the care of a man is not yet complete because eating alone will not keep a man well; he must also exercise. While possessing opposite qualities, food, and exercise work together to produce health.*"

— HIPPOCRATES

These wise words from the "Father of Medicine" himself emphasize a profound truth about our well-being: our health journey is an intricate dance between diet and exercise. I'll tell you why.

Imagine your body as an engine, fueled by the food you eat, and exercise acts as the perfect catalyst, enhancing the efficiency of this engine. This chapter explores this interplay, focusing on the pivotal role of physical exercise and weight management in lowering blood pressure and ameliorating heart health.

This chapter will dive deep into the connection between our bodies' physical exertion and heart health. We'll explore how different forms of exercise contribute to weight management and, consequently, blood pressure control.

GET MOVING

There is an old saying: "A body in motion stays in motion." This principle couldn't be truer when managing high blood pressure. Regular physical activity is not just a recommendation but a necessity, acting as an antidote to hypertension and an elixir for overall heart health. But how does exercise do this?

Exercise aids in lowering blood pressure by enhancing cardiovascular health and boosting the efficiency of our circulatory system. As we move, our heart, the hard-working muscle that it is pumps blood throughout our body more effectively. This efficiency reduces the force on our artery walls, thereby decreasing our blood pressure. It's a simple yet powerful cycle that starts with the decision to get moving.

As we maintain a healthy weight, our blood pressure levels tend to normalize, reducing the likelihood of hypertension and associated health risks. Furthermore, physical activity helps manage other risk factors synonymous with high blood pressure. Take obesity, for example. Regular exercise aids in weight management, reducing the strain on the heart that excess weight often causes.

For those battling diabetes, another risk factor for high blood pressure, exercise is a vital ally. Physical activity aids in regulating blood sugar levels, increasing insulin sensitivity, and promoting a healthier metabolic state. By integrating regular exercise into our routine, we can manage diabetes more effectively, mitigating its impact on our blood pressure.

Stress, a silent contributor to high blood pressure, can be significantly managed through regular exercise. Physical activity releases endorphins, the body's natural mood lifters, promoting well-being and relaxation. This stress reduction can indirectly aid blood pressure control, contributing to our overall heart health.

Now, let's dive into the benefits of exercise on heart health. Regular physical activity strengthens the heart muscle, enabling it to pump blood more efficiently, thereby reducing the pressure on the arteries. This heart-strengthening effect, over time, can lead to a sustainable decrease in resting heart rate and blood pressure.

Exercise also promotes better lipid profiles by raising good cholesterol (HDL) levels and reducing bad cholesterol (LDL) levels. This balance can prevent cholesterol buildup in arteries, reducing the risk of atherosclerosis and heart disease.

Moreover, the increased blood flow during exercise delivers more oxygen and essential nutrients to the tissues, including the heart. This enhanced circulation promotes the healing and growth of the cells, further improving the function and structure of the cardiovascular system.

Physical activity also aids in maintaining a healthy vascular function by improving endothelial function, promoting vascular remodeling, and enhancing baroreflex sensitivity. These changes can further lower blood pressure and contribute to the heart's overall health.

Moreover, when safeguarding heart health, physical activity wears the crown. Its benefits extend far beyond calorie-burning or physique-shaping; it is the linchpin in maintaining optimal cardiovascular health. But what makes regular exercise such a powerful ally for our hearts?

1. The heart is a muscle; like other muscles, it grows stronger with exercise. Regular physical activity enables our heart to pump blood more efficiently throughout the body, reducing the strain on this vital organ. Over time, this lessens the risk of heart disease, including conditions like heart failure.

2. Exercise positively influences blood flow in multiple ways. It helps arteries maintain their elasticity, ensuring smooth, unimpeded blood flow. Enhanced circulation also means more oxygen and vital nutrients are delivered to the body's tissues, leading to better overall health and, specifically, a healthier heart.

3. Regular physical activity helps manage blood lipid levels, namely triglycerides, and cholesterol.

4. Exercise plays a vital role in achieving and maintaining a healthy weight, which is crucial for heart health. Excess weight strains the heart, increasing the risk of hypertension, high cholesterol, and diabetes—all risk factors for heart disease.

5. Regular physical activity helps lower blood pressure, a key benefit for those with hypertension. The heart-friendly effects of exercise extend beyond the workout period,

with blood pressure often remaining lower for several hours post-exercise.

6. Exercise is an effective stressbuster. It stimulates the production of endorphins, the body's natural mood lifters. Less stress translates to lower blood pressure over time, further reducing the risk of heart disease.

7. Regular physical activity improves the body's sensitivity to insulin, reducing the risk of type 2 diabetes—a significant risk factor for heart disease. For those already living with diabetes, exercise helps manage the condition, lessening its impact on heart health.

In essence, the relationship between regular exercise and heart health is symbiotic. Physical activity nourishes our heart, providing the support it needs to function optimally, while our heart, in turn, fuels our ability to stay active, fit, and healthy. It's a beautiful, beneficial cycle, and investment in exercise truly is an investment in a healthier, heart-happy future.

EXERCISE OPTIONS FOR YOU

When it comes to exercise's beneficial effects on blood pressure, patience, and consistency are essential. It typically takes between one to three months of regular exercise to see a tangible impact on blood pressure levels. And these benefits, just like the blooms of a well-tended garden, persist only as long as you continue your exercise regimen.

But what type of exercise works best? Here's the good news: you have options, and they're all advantageous in their own unique ways.

1. Cardiovascular or Aerobic Exercise

This form of exercise, which includes activities like jogging, cycling, swimming, or even brisk walking, primarily targets your heart and lungs. Regular aerobic exercise strengthens your heart, making it more efficient at pumping blood and supplying your body with the oxygen it needs. This helps lower blood pressure and is excellent for overall cardiovascular health.

2. Strength Training

Lifting weights or using resistance bands are examples of strength training. While it might seem more suited for those looking to build muscle, it plays a pivotal role in heart health too. Regular strength training helps reduce body fat, increase lean muscle mass, and burn calories more efficiently. This, in turn, aids in weight management, a key factor in maintaining healthy blood pressure levels.

3. Resistance Training

Like strength training, it involves using weights or resistance bands. However, it also includes exercises that use your body weight (like push-ups or squats). This form of exercise not only builds strength and burns calories, but it can also help improve your resting metabolic rate, aiding in weight control and hence, blood pressure management.

4. Stretching

While stretching may not directly lower blood pressure, it plays a supporting role in your overall exercise regimen. Regular stretching keeps your body flexible and injury-free, allowing you to maintain a consistent exercise routine. Furthermore, practices such as yoga, which include an emphasis on deep breathing and relaxation, can help lower stress levels, a contributing factor to high blood pressure.

Remember, a well-rounded exercise routine comprising cardiovascular exercise, strength training, resistance training, and stretching is the secret recipe to combat high blood pressure and enhance heart health.

The key is to remain consistent, as the fruits of your efforts, although not immediate, will surely be rewarding. Your journey toward a healthier heart is a marathon, not a sprint.

THE ART OF EXERCISING RIGHT

When it comes to exercise, it's not merely about doing it; it's about doing it right. The duration, intensity, and consistency of your exercise routine play pivotal roles in effectively managing blood pressure and promoting overall heart health.

Let's dive into the optimal exercise framework, one that is both beneficial and sustainable.

1. The Gold Standard – 30 Minutes of Moderate Activity

Whether you enjoy brisk walking, a leisurely bike ride, or a spirited dance class, engaging in moderate activity for at least 30 minutes five days a week lays the foundation for a heart-healthy exercise routine. This goal is as pragmatic as it is beneficial, designed to accommodate the busiest of schedules.

2. Short on Time? Intensify!

When time constraints challenge your commitment, don't despair! The beauty of exercise lies in its flexibility. If carving out 30 minutes proves difficult, consider vigorous activities like jogging or high-intensity interval training (HIIT). A focused 20-minute session of such vigorous exercise, three to four days a week, can yield the same heart health benefits as longer, moderate activity sessions.

3. Begin at the Beginning – Gradual Is Good

If you're at the start of your exercise journey, take heart in knowing that every journey begins with a single step. Aim for consistency over intensity initially. Gradually work up to the recommended amount of exercise over a few weeks, respecting your body's pace and limitations.

4. Warming Up – The Prelude to a Safe Workout

A safe and effective workout begins with a warm-up. Consider it the gentle wake-up call that prepares your body for the activity ahead. Start with a 5- to 10-minute warm-up routine that slowly increases your heart rate while loosening your muscles and joints. The key is to increase the intensity gradually; a good gauge is being able to carry on with a conversation while exercising.

5. Cooling Down – An Essential Encore

Exercise is a cycle, and its completion lies in a proper cool-down period. After a workout, take a few minutes to slow down your activity level gradually. This wind-down phase is especially important for individuals with high blood pressure. It allows the heart rate and blood pressure to return to resting levels gradually, reducing strain on the heart.

Ultimately, the perfect exercise routine fits seamlessly into your lifestyle, is enjoyable, and respects your body's needs and limitations. Remember that the true value of exercise lies in its regularity rather than intensity. And like any good habit, the benefits of exercise compound over time. Your commitment today, however small it might seem, is an investment in a healthier, heart-happier future.

STAYING THE COURSE: NURTURING A SUSTAINABLE EXERCISE ROUTINE

Sustaining an exercise routine can be a challenge, especially in our ever-busy lives. Yet, consistency is the lifeblood of a beneficial workout regime. Here are some strategies to help you keep that commitment to your heart's health:

1. Choose an exercise activity that you enjoy. This isn't merely about 'getting fit'; it's about finding joy in movement and creating a space in your day that you look forward to. Whether it's the peace of yoga, the rhythm of dance, or the exhilaration of cycling, make sure it's something that speaks to your spirit.

2. Set realistic, achievable fitness goals. While the overarching goal is heart health, having smaller, measurable objectives can be incredibly motivating. It could be walking an extra kilometer, shaving a minute off your run time, or mastering a new yoga pose. Celebrate these milestones; they are steps on your journey to heart health.

3. Establishing a regular exercise schedule helps transform your workout from a 'to-do' into a habit. If you're a morning person, harness that

energy into an invigorating start to your day. If evenings are your time, wind down with a calming yoga session. Find a rhythm that fits your lifestyle.

4. On days when time is scarce, or energy levels are low, remember that a shorter workout is better than no workout at all. Even a brisk 10-minute walk contributes to your goal. Consistency trumps duration.

5. Engage in physical activities with a partner or a group. Exercising with others can be fun and motivating. It creates a sense of community and accountability, which can help keep you on track.

6. Incorporate variety into your routine to prevent boredom. Try new activities, alternate between different types of exercises, or change your workout environment. Variety keeps your workouts fresh and exciting.

7. Rest when you need to, modify exercises when necessary, and seek professional advice if you have any health concerns. An exercise routine should respect your body's needs and limitations.

Remember, exercise is a celebration of what your body can do, not a punishment for what you eat. Let this perspective guide you in nurturing an exercise routine that enhances not only your heart health but also your overall well-being.

EXERCISE GUIDELINES FOR OLDER ADULTS

Throughout the different stages of life, our bodies undergo a variety of changes. Yet, one constant remains —the importance of physical activity. Regardless of age, exercise plays a vital role in maintaining our health and well-being. However, as we grow older, the approach to fitness necessitates more caution and care, as personal health conditions and capabilities must be prioritized.

Older adults are recommended to engage in at least 150 minutes of moderate-intensity aerobic activity per week, or 75 minutes of vigorous-intensity activity, along with muscle-strengthening activities at least twice weekly. But remember, these are general guide-lines and must be adjusted to individual capacities and health circumstances.

Consultation with a healthcare provider can help design an exercise regimen that respects your specific considerations while optimizing your heart health and overall well-being. For older adults commencing their journey into regular physical activity, the best advice is to start slow. Initiating your fitness regime with low-impact activities like walking is an excellent choice.

Over time, intensity and duration can be gradually increased. Include exercises that promote flexibility, balance, and strength, such as gentle yoga or tai chi in your regimen. Most importantly, listen to your body and remember to rest when required.

Prior to starting or modifying an exercise routine, it's crucial to engage in a detailed conversation with your healthcare provider. Four essential questions should guide this discussion:

1. "What types of exercises would be suitable for me?"

Rationale: This question helps determine what forms of exercise align with your current health status, fitness level, and personal preferences. Everyone is unique, and what works well for one person may not work as well for another. Your healthcare provider can assess your current physical condition and recommend exercises that suit your fitness level. For example, if you have joint problems, low-impact exercises like swimming or cycling might be suitable.

2. "Are there any exercises or activities I should avoid?"

Rationale: Certain health conditions can make specific exercises risky. It's essential to identify these potential issues to prevent unnecessary harm and complications. Depending on your health status, your healthcare provider might advise against certain high-impact or strenuous exercises. For instance, individuals with heart conditions might need to avoid overly intense cardio workouts.

3. "How does my health condition affect my ability to exercise?"

Rationale: Your overall health and any pre-existing conditions can directly influence your capacity to exercise. Certain diseases require particular care and precautions during physical activity. For example, if you have osteoporosis, weight-bearing exercises might be beneficial, but with caution to avoid fractures. If you have diabetes, your provider will advise you on managing blood sugar levels during and after exercise.

4. "Is my preventive care up to date?"

Rationale: Keeping your preventive care up to date ensures you're exercising with the knowledge that any underlying health issues are managed and you're not putting your health at unnecessary risk. Your provider can guide you on any necessary screenings, tests, or vaccinations. For example, if you're at risk for heart disease, regular cholesterol and blood pressure check-ups are crucial.

Remember, these answers should act as a guide, and you should always consult with your healthcare provider for personalized advice. In all scenarios, the primary goal is to engage in physical activity safely and effectively for the betterment of your overall health and well-being.

Understanding which exercises might be limited by certain health conditions can help you avoid unnecessary harm and concentrate on safe and beneficial activities. Additionally, being aware of how specific diseases influence your exercise capacities and precautions enables a tailored fitness approach.

Lastly, ensuring that your preventive screenings and tests are current equips you with the confidence to engage in physical activity, knowing that any underlying health issues are effectively managed. These discussions and considerations are equally important for both genders. Despite men and women facing similar risks due to inactivity, like heart disease, diabetes, and osteoporosis, specific factors like menopause-related changes in women warrant additional attention.

Exercising in the golden years isn't solely about maintaining heart health. It's integral to independence, mood enhancement, and boosting the overall quality of life. With the right guidance and personalized approach, older adults can weave a fitness routine into their lifestyle that truly adds life to their years and years to their life.

OVERCOMING YOUR FEARS

Beginning an exercise routine or reintroducing physical activity into your life can be a daunting endeavor, particularly when you're grappling with uncertainties and fears. It's normal to have apprehensions, but it's crucial not to let these fears stop you from embracing a healthier lifestyle. Let's confront these seven common fitness fears and explore how to conquer them:

1. The Fear of Beginning after a Long Hiatus

If it's been a long while since you last engaged in regular exercise, the idea of starting might feel over-whelming. To conquer this fear, start small and gradu-ally build up. Choose low-impact activities like walking or swimming that are easy on your joints and don't require special skills. It's important to remember that every journey begins with a single step, and it's perfectly okay to start slow and progress at your own pace.

2. The Fear of Lifting Weights

Weightlifting can be intimidating, especially if you're new to it or concerned about the risk of injury. But strength training is crucial for maintaining muscle mass and bone density, especially as we age. Start with light weights or resistance bands and gradually increase the resistance as your strength improves. Consider hiring a personal trainer or joining a group class for beginners to learn proper techniques.

3. The Fear of Falling

The fear of falling and injuring oneself is valid, particu-larly for older adults. Balance exercises and strength training can help reduce this fear by improving your stability and coordination. Tai chi and yoga are excellent choices for enhancing balance. Use supportive equipment like handrails or exercise machines to maintain stability if needed.

4. The Fear of Inducing a Heart Attack

While it's true that physical exertion can stress the heart, the right kind and amount of exercise are beneficial for cardiovascular health. Start with moderate activities and increase your intensity gradually. Ensure that you're cleared by your doctor before starting an exercise regimen, especially if you have a history of heart disease.

5. The Fear of Exacerbating Joint Pain

It's a common misconception that exercise will make joint pain worse. In reality, regular, low-impact activities can help alleviate joint pain by strengthening the muscles around the joints and enhancing flexibility. Consider exercises like swimming, biking, or water aerobics, which are gentle on the knees.

6. The Fear of Disrupting Blood Sugar Control

Physical activity can indeed influence blood sugar levels. However, with proper management, exercise is highly beneficial for people with diabetes. Monitor your blood sugar levels before and after exercise and make the necessary adjustments to your meals or medication with your doctor's guidance.

7. The Fear of Being Too Weak, Old, or Disabled

Age or disability should not preclude you from exercising. Everyone, irrespective of age, ability, or health status can benefit from physical activity. Adapt the exercise to your abilities—seated or low-impact exercises can be effective options. Remember to consult with healthcare professionals or physiotherapists who can help design a safe and suitable exercise plan for you.

Ultimately, these fears, while valid, should not impede your journey toward better health. Start slow, seek professional guidance, listen to your body, and gradually push your boundaries. Fitness is not a destination but a way of life, and it's never too late to start living healthily.

BUILDING A COMMUNITY

"The best way to keep your blood pressure down is to know what makes it go up."

— MEISTER JOHANSEN

I'd like to ask you to take a moment to think about how you felt when you first received your diagnosis.

What emotions were running through you? Were you scared? Anxious? Overwhelmed? Did you ask yourself where you went wrong or if this was all your fault?

These are all common reactions to receiving a diagnosis of high blood pressure, and I've witnessed countless patients experience them. Suddenly being faced with a lifetime of monitoring and medication is overwhelming, and it can make you feel very isolated – even though you know that many other people are living with the condition.

This is why I'm committed to supporting as many people as possible – and to help me do that, I'd like to ask you to get involved.

The good news is, doing so will barely make a dent in your schedule, and you don't even have to leave your chair. All I'd like you to do is leave a review.

By leaving a review of this book on Amazon, you'll help other people living with high blood pressure feel less alone and point them in the direction of the support and guidance they're looking for.

Simply by telling new readers how this book has helped you and what they'll find inside, you'll help me to provide support for more people.

Thank you so much for your help. We can't reverse that feeling someone gets when they first receive their diagnosis, but we can help them to take control going forward. Together, we can build a community.

Scan to Leave a Review!

6

REST AND RELAXATION

W hile it is commonplace to hear about the importance of diet and exercise in controlling blood pressure and safeguarding our heart health, we often overlook two other crucial contributors: quality sleep and effective stress management. Though silent in their operation, these invisible architects of health are powerful in their impact.

The old adage that "Sleep is the best meditation" by the Dalai Lama captures the essence of what this chapter aims to explore. Like a dedicated night-shift worker, quality sleep silently rejuvenates us, repairs our bodies, and prepares us for the battles of the next day. At the same time, effective stress management ensures our emotional armor is ever ready to deal with life's challenges.

In this chapter, we will delve into the intricacies of these critical health components, unraveling their direct and indirect impacts on blood pressure levels. As I uncover the mechanics of restful sleep and the power of keeping stress in check, I'll provide practical, actionable steps that you can incorporate into your daily routines.

Embracing the trifecta of quality sleep, restful breaks, and nurturing tranquility forms a robust defense line in the fight against hypertension. Each component serves as a unique piece of the puzzle that, when combined, boosts your overall heart health. During sleep, our bodies and minds embark on a silent yet essential mission of restoration.

This undisturbed period of rest allows us to mend from the day's wear and tear, leading to a refreshing dawn. However, sleep's elusiveness or insufficiency can set off a chain reaction, increasing stress hormones that may elevate blood pressure and give rise to additional health concerns. Therefore, fostering a sleep environment conducive to restful nights becomes necessary for healthy living.

Interlacing moments of serenity within our day is another key to managing blood pressure. Methods may vary from deep breathing exercises to meditation or simply immersing oneself in a calming hobby. These practices aid in lowering stress levels, effectively serving as an antidote to the constant barrage of life's challenges.

Chronic stress, an often silent but destructive force, is linked to high blood pressure and other health complications. Therefore, like a skilled sailor steering through stormy seas, the ability to keep stress in check becomes an essential skill. Implementing effective stress management techniques aids in sustaining balanced blood pressure levels, contributing to your heart's longevity. By intertwining adequate sleep, moments of calm, and stress management, we build a resilient bulwark for our heart health.

SLEEP

Sleep: It's a universal experience yet cloaked in a veil of mystery. It's a fascinating biological process that scientists are still fervently unraveling. But what is sleep exactly, and why is it so important? Let's dive into this nocturnal world that holds the key to our health and well-being.

Sleep is a natural, recurring state of mind and body characterized by altered consciousness, relatively inhibited sensory activity, reduced interactions with surroundings, and a complex ballet of brain activities.

This state is divided into two overarching categories: Rapid Eye Movement (REM) sleep and Non-REM sleep.

Non-REM sleep is further classified into three stages. The first stage represents the bridge from wakefulness to sleep, a period of light sleep when our heartbeat, breathing, and eye movements slow down. The second stage sees the continued slowing of these physiological processes along with brain waves, with occasional bursts of electrical activity. The third stage, often called deep sleep, is vital for feeling refreshed and revitalized the next day.

REM sleep, occurring approximately 90 minutes after falling asleep, is marked by rapid eye movements, increased respiration rate, and brain activity. It's during this stage that vivid dreaming often occurs. These sleep stages form a cycle that repeats multiple times during the night, each stage playing a unique role in the physical and mental rejuvenation process.

The importance of sleep cannot be overstated. It's during this precious time that the body embarks on essential maintenance work. Tissues are repaired, muscles are rebuilt, and hormones are regulated. It's also during sleep that the brain processes and consolidates memories, flushes out toxins, and recharges for the coming day.

The mechanisms of sleep involve an intricate dance between various regions of the brain, hormones, and neurotransmitters. The hypothalamus, a small region at the base of the brain, houses clusters of nerve cells that act as control centers affecting sleep and arousal. Interactions between these nerve cells, hormones such as melatonin, and neurotransmitters like GABA and glycine, all contribute to the timing, quality, and depth of our sleep.

In summary, sleep is an essential biological function with complex stages and mechanisms. It plays a pivotal role in maintaining physical health, cognitive function, and emotional well-being. Understanding the significance of sleep, its stages, and its mechanisms can provide insight into how we can better prioritize and optimize this vital component of our lives.

Sleep and heart health share an intricate and profound relationship that underscores the vital importance of obtaining quality rest. Indeed, when we surrender ourselves to the night, we don't merely drift into a realm of dreams; we also step into a crucial phase of cardiovascular restoration and repair.

Sleep provides a unique window for our heart to ease its ceaseless work. During quality sleep, our heart rate and blood pressure significantly drop, giving our cardiovascular system a much-needed break. This restorative period also offers the opportunity for the heart and vascular system to repair any damage caused by the day's stressors.

Additionally, healthy sleep patterns can promote improved cholesterol levels and reduce inflammation, both of which are paramount in maintaining heart health and minimizing the risk of cardiovascular diseases.

On the flip side, poor sleep or sleep disorders like sleep apnea can have deleterious effects on heart function. These issues can lead to irregular heartbeat, higher blood pressure, increased inflammation, and elevated stress hormones. Such effects do not only put a strain on the heart but can also increase the risk of heart diseases like hypertension, stroke, and heart failure.

In essence, a good night's sleep is not just a luxury—it's a necessity for a healthy heart and a healthier life.

Sleep problems and heart diseases

Sleep isn't merely a passive, restorative state—it's an intricate physiological process that, when disrupted, can have far-reaching implications for cardiovascular health. Various sleep disorders and irregularities have been associated with an increased risk of heart disease, and this connection becomes even more significant as we age.

Sleep apnea, characterized by episodes of halted breathing during sleep, is a common disorder that disrupts the quality of sleep. This condition can cause sudden drops in blood oxygen levels, leading to increased blood pressure and strain on the cardiovascular system, raising the risk of heart disease and stroke.

Moreover, insomnia, a condition where individuals struggle to fall or stay asleep, can lead to chronic sleep deprivation. This lack of sleep may raise stress hormones, increase blood pressure, and stimulate inflammation, creating a conducive environment for heart disease.

As we age, changes in our sleep architecture become evident. Older individuals often experience a reduction in deep (REM) sleep, encounter more frequent awakenings, and may find it harder to fall asleep. Several factors contribute to these shifts, including changes in circadian rhythm, lifestyle alterations, and health conditions often associated with aging.

Changes in circadian rhythms, our internal biological clock regulating sleep-wake cycles, can lead to earlier sleep and wake times. Lifestyle alterations, such as retirement, can disrupt previous sleep schedules. Moreover, health issues like chronic pain, prostate enlargement, or menopausal symptoms can lead to frequent nighttime awakenings.

These age-related sleep disruptions can further exacerbate the risks of sleep disorders, which can, in turn, negatively impact heart health. Given these complexities, understanding and addressing sleep issues becomes even more critical as we age, not only for heart health but for overall well-being.

As we age, our susceptibility to certain sleep irregularities, which can negatively impact the quality of our slumber and brain oxygen levels, increases. One such notable condition is sleep apnea, marked by distinctive symptoms such as pronounced snoring, intermittent pauses in breathing while asleep, and a pervasive sense of fatigue during the day.

These symptoms don't just disrupt a peaceful night's sleep but also have far-reaching consequences for overall health. One significant aspect relates to the drop in oxygen levels in the brain that occurs during the pauses in breathing, which can result in a host of neurological and cognitive issues.

Furthermore, the disturbances caused by sleep apnea can trigger a cascade of physiological responses. Each episode of halted breathing jolts the body from deep sleep to a lighter stage or even full wakefulness, preventing restorative sleep stages that are key for cognitive functions and physical recovery.

Sleep apnea has also been recognized as a major contributor to hypertension, a topic addressed in an earlier chapter. The repeated oxygen deprivation and subsequent recovery periods lead to increased heart rate and a spike in blood pressure levels, exerting undue stress on the cardiovascular system. Over time, this chronic stress can result in sustained high blood pressure, even during waking hours, amplifying the risk of heart-related complications.

Importantly, the link between sleep apnea and high blood pressure remains robust regardless of other potential contributing factors. Hence, as we grow older, understanding and managing conditions like sleep apnea becomes critical in the pursuit of maintaining not only restful sleep but also long-term cardiovascular health.

Tips for improving sleep

1. **Embrace the Daylight**: Harness the power of natural light during daytime hours. Bright light exposure helps maintain your body's circadian

rhythm, the natural internal process that regulates your sleep-wake cycle.

2. **Evening Blue Light Curfew**: Limit your exposure to blue light—emitted by digital screens and artificial lighting—in the evening. This type of light can interfere with your circadian rhythm and the production of melatonin, a hormone that signals your body when it's time to sleep.

3. **Caffeine Curfew**: Avoid consuming caffeinated beverages later in the day. Caffeine can stay elevated in your blood for 6–8 hours, potentially disrupting your sleep if consumed late.

4. **Nap Mindfully**: While daytime naps can be refreshing, long or irregular napping can negatively impact your nighttime sleep quality. If you must nap, keep it short and consistent.

5. **Consistency Is Key**: Try to maintain a regular sleep schedule, going to bed and waking up at the same time each day. This habit can enhance sleep quality by aligning your sleep routine with your body's internal clock.

6. **Alcohol Abstention**: Alcohol can interfere with your sleep cycle and the quality of your sleep, making you more likely to wake up during the night.

7. **Create a Sleep Haven**: Your bedroom environment significantly impacts your ability to fall asleep. Factors such as noise, light, and furniture arrangement should be optimized for sleep.

8. **Cool It Down**: Experiment with different temperatures to find the setting that suits you best. Most people sleep best in a cooler room.

9. **Dinner Timing**: Avoid heavy meals late in the evening. Your body needs time to digest before sleep, and a full stomach can keep you awake.

10. **Evening Relaxation**: Incorporate calming activities into your evening routine. Techniques like meditation, deep breathing, or gentle yoga can help relax your mind and prepare your body for sleep.

11. **The Power of Warmth**: Consider a relaxing bath or shower before bed. The rise and subsequent fall in body temperature can promote feelings of drowsiness.

12. **Assess Your Sleep Health**: If you consistently have difficulty sleeping, you may have a sleep disorder. Consult a healthcare professional for a proper evaluation.

13. **Invest in Comfort**: Your bed, mattress, and pillow play a significant role in sleep quality.

Prioritize comfort and proper support to ensure the best sleep possible.

14. **Move Your Body**: Regular physical activity can help you sleep better. However, try to avoid strenuous workouts close to bedtime as they can interfere with sleep.

15. **Liquid Limitation**: Drinking liquids before bed can lead to disruptive middle-of-the-night trips to the bathroom. Try to minimize your intake in the hours leading up to bedtime.

STRESS MANAGEMENT

Stress is a universal human experience, a psychological and physiological response to life's demands, challenges, and pressures. It's your body's way of protecting you and responding to any kind of demand or threat, essentially a 'fight or flight' response to perceived danger. However, when this response is chronically activated, it can have detrimental effects on your health, including on your heart and blood pressure.

Stress hormones like adrenaline and cortisol are released into your bloodstream when you encounter a stressful situation. These hormones cause an increase in heart rate, a surge in energy, and a narrowing of the blood vessels—all mechanisms designed for survival during a perceived threat.

Unfortunately, repeated or chronic stress can keep these physiological changes activated, leading to persistently high blood pressure, also known as hypertension. Hypertension is a significant risk factor for heart disease and stroke, among other complications.

So, how can we manage stress to control blood pressure better? The answer lies in a combination of lifestyle modifications, relaxation techniques, and healthy coping strategies. Here are a few practical steps:

1. **Mind-Body Practices**: Techniques like meditation, yoga, and deep-breathing exercises can help reduce stress by calming the mind and relaxing the body. Regular practice can help lower the heart rate and blood pressure, promoting overall heart health.
2. **Physical Activity**: Regular exercise releases endorphins, the body's natural mood lifters. It also helps to lower blood pressure by making your heart stronger and more efficient at pumping blood.
3. **Balanced Diet**: Consuming a balanced diet rich in fruits, vegetables, lean protein, and whole grains can keep your body nourished and equipped to handle stress.
4. **Restful Sleep**: Quality sleep is crucial for stress management. Sleep helps your brain function

properly and regulate mood, improving your ability to cope with stress.

5. **Positive Social Interactions**: Engaging in social activities, spending time with loved ones, or interacting with a supportive community can provide emotional relief and decrease feelings of stress.

6. **Professional Help**: If stress continues to be overwhelming, consider seeking help from a professional. Therapists or counselors trained in stress management can provide tools and techniques tailored to your unique situation.

7. **Relaxation Techniques**: Progressive muscle relaxation, guided imagery, and biofeedback are techniques that can help you control your body's response to stress, helping to lower blood pressure.

8. **Time Management**: Managing your time effectively can help reduce feelings of pressure and overwhelm, thereby mitigating stress.

9. **Positive Mindset**: Maintaining a positive outlook, practicing gratitude, and employing mindfulness can help counter the negative mental and physical effects of stress.

Stress is an inescapable part of life, but its impact on your health is largely within your control. By identifying stress triggers and developing healthy coping strategies, you can manage stress effectively, promote healthier blood pressure levels, and foster overall well-being. Remember, everyone is different, and it's crucial to find a stress management approach that works for you.

Techniques to reduce stress

Understanding and implementing stress reduction techniques is an essential step toward better overall health. These strategies can help mitigate the effects of stress, particularly its impact on blood pressure levels. Let's explore six such techniques:

1. Breathing Techniques

Deep, focused breathing exercises are quick and effective stress relievers. They work by activating your body's natural relaxation response, slowing your heart rate, and lowering your blood pressure. Simply inhaling deeply through your nose, holding your breath for a few seconds, and then exhaling slowly through your mouth can have a calming effect.

2. Physical Exercise

Regular physical activity is a powerful stress reducer. It promotes the release of endorphins, your body's natural mood boosters. Moreover, it also helps lower blood pressure by improving heart health and enhancing circulation. Choose an exercise routine that you enjoy, whether it's walking, swimming, dancing, or cycling, and try to incorporate it into your daily schedule.

3. Mindfulness

This is the practice of staying fully present in the moment, observing your thoughts and feelings without judgment. Mindfulness can be cultivated through various activities like meditation, mindful eating, or even simple mindful breathing. Practicing mindfulness can help decrease stress by fostering a greater sense of calm and awareness.

4. Progressive Muscle Relaxation

This involves gradually tensing and then relaxing each muscle group in your body, starting from your toes, and working your way up to your head. It's an effective technique for reducing physical tension and mental stress, helping you to feel more relaxed and in control.

5. Visualization

Also known as guided imagery, visualization involves forming peaceful and positive mental images to replace negative or stressful thoughts. Envisioning a tranquil place or scenario can help soothe your mind and body, reducing stress and promoting relaxation.

6. Yoga

Combining physical postures, breathing exercises, and meditation, yoga is an excellent practice for stress management. Regular yoga practice can improve your body's physical response to stress, promoting lower blood pressure, enhanced relaxation, and mental tranquility.

These techniques not only help in mitigating stress but also contribute to the overall sense of well-being. Integrating them into your lifestyle can lead to better blood pressure control, improved emotional health, and enhanced resilience to life's challenges. Remember, consistency is key; make these practices a part of your regular routine to reap their full benefits.

Ways to reduce stress with therapy

Therapeutic methods of stress reduction can add an enjoyable and creative dimension to your stress management regimen. Incorporating these therapies into your lifestyle can offer a holistic approach to maintaining balanced blood pressure levels. Let's explore four such therapies:

1. Aromatherapy

Utilizing aromatic essential oils, aromatherapy can create a calming environment and stimulate the senses, providing relief from stress. Certain scents like lavender, bergamot, or ylang-ylang have been found particularly effective in promoting relaxation. Whether used in diffusers, body oils, or during a bath, the fragrance of these oils can soothe your mind and foster tranquility.

2. Art Therapy

This form of therapy uses the creative process of making art to improve mental well-being. Artistic expression, be it painting, drawing, sculpting, or any other medium, can be a powerful outlet for stress and can help you channel emotions constructively. It doesn't require you to be an artist; the focus is on the process, not the final product.

3. Massage Therapy

A well-executed massage can work wonders in alleviating physical tension and promoting relaxation. By manipulating the body's soft tissues, massage can improve circulation, ease muscle tension, and enhance feelings of overall well-being, thereby helping to mitigate stress-induced blood pressure spikes.

4. Music Therapy

Music has a profound impact on our emotions and can be a potent tool for stress management. Whether you're playing an instrument, singing, or just listening to soothing tunes, music therapy can lower stress levels, reduce heart rate, and create a serene mindset. Choose the type of music that resonates with you, as personal preference plays a significant role in the effectiveness of music therapy.

Exploring these therapeutic avenues to alleviate stress can be rewarding and enjoyable. They provide a multifaceted approach to stress management, helping you find your unique path toward calmness and equanimity, thereby supporting healthier blood pressure levels. Remember, it's not just about reducing stress; it's about enhancing your quality of life and finding joy in the journey.

As we've underscored throughout, securing restful sleep, and effectively navigating stress are key to sustaining optimal blood pressure levels. That said, other lifestyle habits like smoking and alcohol intake can significantly influence your blood pressure.

Consequently, the next chapter will delve deeper into how these behaviors impact blood pressure. We'll also take a look at some useful advice on mitigating or completely ceasing these habits for the sake of enhancing your cardiovascular well-being.

7

KICKING BAD HABITS

"**M**ost people don't have that willingness to break bad habits. They have a lot of excuses, and they talk like victims."

— CARLOS SANTANA

There exist two lifestyle habits that often lurk in the shadow of health discussions—smoking and alcohol consumption. These behaviors can significantly impact blood pressure levels, often escalating them into unhealthy ranges.

In this chapter, I intend to illuminate the intricate links between these habits and heart health, along with a detailed look at the potential effects of these habits on blood pressure. My focus will be on helping you understand these connections and offering practical, actionable, guidance to curtail or completely stop these habits, setting the stage for an improved cardiovascular health landscape.

As Carlos Santana aptly pointed out, breaking free from detrimental habits is often a daunting challenge. People tend to cradle their vices, swaddling them in layers of reasons and perceived helplessness.

Yet, the true essence of self-improvement resides in the courage to acknowledge our weaknesses and the determination to transform them. The path of transformation, however, isn't devoid of hardships. We can easily fall prey to the soothing whispers of excuses, rendering us mere victims in our own narratives. Yet, we must remember that no improvement was ever won by comfort alone. The change that begets improvement is often uncomfortable, sometimes painful, but always worthwhile.

Take smoking and excessive alcohol consumption, for example. They are often clung onto as coping mechanisms, means of socialization, or simply out of habitual routine. However, they wield a double-edged sword, offering momentary relief or pleasure at the expense of long-term health—specifically cardiovascular health.

Asserting control over one's health is a fundamental duty incumbent upon each of us. Instead of merely leaning on the guidance of healthcare practitioners to regulate your well-being, it is vital to initiate an active stance toward self-care. Shaking off detrimental behaviors such as smoking and excessive indulgence in alcohol is an exercise in self-responsibility and self-regulation.

Acknowledging the profound influence these habits can exert on our health and wellness is a critical aspect of managing elevated blood pressure and circumventing associated health complications. Overcoming these ingrained habits can indeed be a Herculean task, but the active pursuit of curbing or discontinuing smoking, along with curtailing alcohol consumption, is nonnegotiable. This implies being answerable for our choices and understanding the significant impact our habits imprint on our comprehensive health status.

SMOKING CESSATION

Smoking cessation is a crucial step toward a healthier life, and its positive impact on blood pressure cannot be overstated. The question that often arises is: "How does smoking elevate blood pressure?" The nicotine in cigarettes stimulates the body to produce adrenaline, which in turn increases heart rate and narrows blood vessels.

The result is a temporary spike in blood pressure every time a person smokes.

In the long term, smoking can damage blood vessels, reducing their elasticity and making them more prone to accumulate fatty deposits leading to atherosclerosis —a major risk factor for high blood pressure. Deciding to quit smoking brings immediate and long-term benefits for blood pressure management and overall heart health.

Within 20 minutes of stubbing out the last cigarette, the heart rate and blood pressure begin to normalize. Over the subsequent hours and days, carbon monoxide levels in the blood drop, and oxygen levels rise, improving blood circulation and reducing the strain on the heart.

Several weeks after quitting, the risk of heart attack starts to decline. After about a year, the excess risk of coronary heart disease is half that of a smoker. Over the course of 5 to 15 years, the risk of stroke also reduces to that of a nonsmoker.

Furthermore, quitting smoking can lead to an improvement in blood pressure, often within a few days. This is primarily due to the elimination of the immediate effects of nicotine on blood pressure and heart rate. The extent to which blood pressure drops after quitting smoking can vary depending on individual health circumstances and lifestyle factors, but even a small decrease can have a significant impact on cardiovascular health.

It's important to note, however, that while quitting smoking can lead to an immediate reduction in blood pressure, it does not reverse any damage that has already been done to the blood vessels. Therefore, individuals who have smoked for many years, or who have other risk factors for high blood pressure, should continue to monitor their blood pressure regularly and take steps to maintain a heart-healthy lifestyle.

In essence, cessation of smoking is one of the most impactful actions one can take for one's heart health, and while the journey may be challenging, the rewards are immeasurable. With the right support and commitment, quitting smoking can be a significant stride toward a healthier life, characterized by better blood pressure control and a lower risk of heart disease.

Steps to quit smoking

Embracing the journey to quit smoking involves setting clear goals, planning meticulously, and executing your plan with determination. Here are nine thoughtful steps to guide you through this process:

1. **Establish Your "Quit Day" and Commit**: Begin by setting a specific date as your "Quit Day." This day signifies your commitment to a smoke-free life. As part of this commitment, take a No Smoking pledge—a powerful, personal affirmation of your resolve to quit smoking.

2. **Decide Your Quitting Strategy**: There are different strategies to quit smoking, and you need to choose one that aligns with your habits and preferences. You could quit cold turkey, which means abruptly stopping without any aids, or you could gradually reduce your smoking frequency until you stop entirely. Alternatively, you could choose to smoke only a part of each cigarette, gradually reducing the amount until you quit completely.

3. **Consult a Healthcare Professional**: Schedule an appointment with your doctor or a healthcare provider. They can provide useful advice and might recommend medicines or support programs that can increase your chances of quitting successfully.

4. **Craft Your Quitting Plan**: Prior to your Quit Day, make a detailed plan that outlines your strategy. This could include tactics to handle

cravings, cues to remind you why you're quitting, and rewards for reaching milestones.

5. **Stock Up on Healthy Snacks**: Combat nicotine cravings with healthy snacks. Foods like fruits, nuts, and yogurt can not only help distract you from smoking but also contribute to a healthier lifestyle.

6. **Discover Engaging Distractions**: Identify enjoyable activities to keep you occupied during the times you're usually tempted to smoke. These could include hobbies, exercise, reading, or even puzzles.

7. **Purge Smoking Triggers**: Eliminate any reminder of smoking from your environment. Discard all cigarettes, matches, lighters, ashtrays, and any other tobacco products from your home, office, and car. A clean environment can support your clean break from smoking.

8. **Quit Tobacco on Your Quit Day**: When the day arrives, commit wholeheartedly to your decision. Stick to your plan, lean on your support systems, and remember why you chose to quit.

ALCOHOL CONSUMPTION

While occasional indulgence in a glass of wine, beer, or a favorite cocktail can be part of a balanced lifestyle, it's imperative to remain mindful of the quantity consumed to maintain optimal health. Excessive alcohol intake can lead to detrimental health effects, including the disruption of your cardiovascular system, particularly your blood pressure.

Alcohol has the ability to temporarily increase blood pressure levels, and when consumed in excess over a prolonged period, it can lead to sustained hypertension. The reason lies in the nature of alcohol itself: it is a vasodilator, which means it causes blood vessels to relax and widen. While this might initially seem like it would lower blood pressure, the body counteracts this effect by constricting the blood vessels, leading to an increase in blood pressure.

The recommended daily alcohol intake varies between genders due to physiological differences. For men, it's suggested to limit alcohol consumption to one to two standard drinks per day, whereas, for women, it's advised to stick to one standard drink per day. A standard drink, as defined in the U.S., typically contains about 14 grams of pure alcohol, which equates to 5 ounces of wine, 12 ounces of beer, or 1.5 ounces of distilled spirits.

Remember, these guidelines are averages, not hard-and-fast rules, and individual tolerance and health impact can vary. It's always crucial to listen to your body and consult with healthcare professionals if you're unsure about your alcohol consumption. Balancing enjoyment with moderation is key to maintaining a healthy lifestyle and ensuring that your heart health isn't compromised by overindulgence.

Beers tend to have a lower alcohol concentration than wines, which in turn are generally less potent than distilled spirits. Therefore, the impact on blood pressure can vary depending on the type of drink consumed, and one must consider this when determining what constitutes 'moderate' drinking.

Alcohol can have a direct influence on blood pressure. At intoxicating levels, it will cause vasodilation but at higher levels; it will trigger the release of certain hormones that constrict blood vessels. This will lead to an immediate increase in blood pressure. While this effect is temporary in moderate drinkers, in heavy drinkers, this can result in a sustained elevation of blood pressure, leading to hypertension.

There are specific groups of individuals for whom even moderate alcohol consumption can be harmful. For instance, people diagnosed with certain heart conditions, such as heart rhythm abnormalities or heart failure, should refrain from alcohol intake.

Alcohol can interfere with the normal functioning of the heart and exacerbate these conditions. For instance, in the case of heart rhythm abnormalities, alcohol can trigger episodes of arrhythmia, particularly atrial fibrillation, a condition characterized by an irregular and often rapid heart rate. In the case of heart failure, alcohol can further weaken the heart muscle, impairing its ability to pump blood efficiently.

While the occasional drink may not be harmful to most individuals, it's crucial to understand the potential risks associated with alcohol consumption, especially for those with underlying health conditions.

Consultation with a healthcare professional is highly recommended to determine individual risk factors and set guidelines for safe drinking habits. Maintaining moderation and being mindful of your alcohol intake is a significant step toward preserving cardiovascular health and maintaining healthy blood pressure levels.

Tips on reducing alcohol consumption

Walking on the journey to reduce or eliminate alcohol consumption is a significant commitment to your health. Here are some practical steps to help you along the way:

1. **Put It in Writing**: The first step toward change is often the articulation of your intention. Write down your goal to reduce or stop alcohol consumption. Writing it down gives it a tangible form and serves as a constant reminder of your commitment.

2. **Set a Drinking Goal**: Define what moderation means for you. Decide on the number of days in a week you want to be alcohol-free and the maximum number of drinks you'll have on the days you do consume alcohol.

3. **Keep a Diary of Your Drinking**: Monitoring your consumption can help you recognize patterns and identify triggers. It can provide insights into when and why you drink, which can inform your strategies for reducing consumption.

4. **Empty Your House**: To avoid unnecessary temptation, don't keep alcohol in your home. This ensures that it's not easily accessible,

which can significantly help in the initial stages of reducing consumption.

5. **Drink Slowly**: When you do drink, savor it. Take small sips and make a single drink last. This can help reduce the overall quantity consumed.

6. **Choose Alcohol-Free Days**: Dedicate specific days each week when you will abstain from drinking altogether. This helps you break habitual drinking patterns.

7. **Watch for Peer Pressure**: Be mindful of social situations where you might feel pressured to drink. Have a plan to politely decline or opt for nonalcoholic beverages instead.

8. **Keep Busy:** Engage in activities that you enjoy, and that keep you occupied, reducing the likelihood of reaching for a drink out of boredom or habit.

9. **Ask for Support**: Share your goal with trusted friends and family. Their understanding and encouragement can provide a crucial support system as you navigate this journey.

10. **Guard Against Temptation**: Avoid situations where you might be tempted to drink excessively. This could mean opting for social activities that don't revolve around alcohol.

11. **Be Persistent**: Remember, progress is rarely a straight line. There may be setbacks, but don't let them deter you. Persistence is key to achieving your goal.

Reducing or eliminating alcohol consumption is a personal journey and may require tailored strategies based on individual circumstances. Remember, it's okay to seek professional help if you're finding it difficult to manage on your own. Health professionals can provide the necessary support and resources to ensure your success.

As we reach the conclusion of this chapter, we have unraveled the profound influences that smoking and alcohol consumption exert on blood pressure levels. Now, as we turn the page, we're about to delve into another fascinating dimension of heart health—the realm of complementary and alternative interventions.

These strategies can provide additional support in our pursuit of optimal heart health, enhancing your understanding and widening the array of tools we have at our disposal. Stay tuned as we explore this further in the upcoming chapter.

8

BEYOND MEDICATIONS

I n this chapter, we embark on a journey to explore the diverse world of complementary and alternative interventions designed to manage blood pressure levels. Just like supporting actors in a play who, though not in the limelight, significantly contribute to the play's success, dietary supplements can offer supportive roles in the pursuit of heart health. They may not be the primary characters in the narrative of managing high blood pressure, yet they contribute substantially to the broader ensemble cast promoting cardiovascular well-being.

Supplements often serve as an adjunct to conventional therapies, adding an extra layer of support. They can provide essential nutrients and substances that our bodies need, supplementing our diet and enhancing our body's natural ability to maintain healthy blood pressure levels.

Keep in mind that supplements are not meant to replace prescribed medication or a healthy lifestyle, but rather complement these primary approaches. This is important because addressing high blood pressure often demands a multi-faceted approach. One that encompasses modifications in lifestyle, the use of prescribed medicines, and other interventions aimed at efficiently reducing blood pressure.

While complementary therapies might not be the frontline defense against high blood pressure, their potential to bolster and synergize with conventional treatments is substantial. Navigating the landscape of high blood pressure management involves harnessing the power of tried-and-tested medical treatments while also leveraging the benefits of supplementary approaches.

Though not a cure in their own right, these complementary measures act as vital pieces in a health puzzle, working in synergy with conventional treatments to create a well-rounded, personalized health plan. Various complementary therapies offer unique advantages, but they all share a common objective: to cultivate an environment that fosters optimal heart health. They provide added value through stress alleviation, nutritional enhancement, and overall wellness improvement.

The goal isn't to upend traditional medical advice or replace prescribed treatments but rather to bolster them. In doing so, we aim to create a more balanced and effective route toward improved heart health.

Moreover, everyone's health journey is distinct, with the ideal blend of treatments being influenced by individual health conditions, personal situations, and preferences. Keeping this in mind, we'll delve into an array of complementary and alternative methods that you might consider integrating into your blood pressure management regimen.

As we delve deeper into this chapter, we'll explore various dietary supplements, their roles, and the evidence backing their efficacy in supporting heart health. Let us journey together into this promising aspect of holistic health management, broadening our understanding of how these supportive actors can help us achieve a healthy and harmonious lifestyle.

OVERVIEW OF COMPLEMENTARY AND ALTERNATIVE THERAPIES

While the phrases "complementary medicine" and "alternative medicine" are frequently used inter-changeably and are both encapsulated in the acronym CAM, signifying Complementary and Alternative Medicine, they have distinct meanings. Each term pertains to practices such as herbal treatments or acupuncture, which lie outside conventional Western medicine. However, they differ in how they're utilized.

Complementary medicine refers to the scenario where unconventional therapies are used in conjunction with, or as a complement to, standard Western medicine. The aim is to enhance the effects of traditional treatments, not to replace them.

For instance, meditation, yoga, or acupuncture may be used alongside prescribed medications and a healthy lifestyle to manage blood pressure. The purpose of these complementary methods is to supplement traditional methods, thereby enhancing their effectiveness and offering additional health benefits. They serve as tools that can boost overall well-being, improve stress management, and aid in lifestyle adjustments necessary for controlling blood pressure.

On the other hand, alternative medicine is employed in lieu of traditional medical practices. Instead of utilizing conventional treatments, individuals might opt for these alternative approaches as their primary health-care strategy. It's essential to understand this distinction to accurately navigate and discuss these healthcare options.

According to Miller (2021), "CAM is frequently seen as bad science but good medicine," illuminates the contrasting views surrounding Complementary and Alternative Medicine. This dichotomy points to the reality that even though these treatments may not always meet the rigorous scientific scrutiny customary in conventional medicine, they often offer valuable benefits to personal health and wellness.

From the lens of rigorous scientific study, CAM therapies are often viewed with a degree of uncertainty. This doubt primarily arises because these practices haven't always undergone the rigorous, large-scale, and double-blind trials that are the gold standard in conventional medical research. Thus, the label "bad science" may be attributed to the perceived deficiency of rigorous scientific evidence supporting these therapies.

However, from the perspective of holistic and patient-focused healthcare, CAM practices are frequently recognized as "good medicine." These therapies aim to enhance health holistically, focusing on the entire individual rather than just the disease. They address various aspects of health, including lifestyle, mental and emotional well-being, and other components contributing to total health. Despite the absence of robust scientific validation, many people have experienced health improvements and an enhanced sense of well-being through these practices.

Thus, while it's essential to scrutinize CAM therapies critically, it's equally crucial to acknowledge their potential merits within a comprehensive approach to healthcare. It's always recommended to consult with a healthcare professional before incorporating any CAM therapies to ensure they align with individual health needs and safety requirements.

MIND-BODY THERAPY

Meditation

Meditation is a time-honored practice that is rooted in various traditions across the world. It is a technique focused on bringing tranquility to the mind and the body by concentrating on a single thought, object, or process, such as breathing. This practice has evolved over centuries and today exists in various forms, each with its unique method but sharing the common goal of attaining inner peace and relaxation.

It's intriguing to note how this seemingly simple mind-body practice can impact physical health parameters, specifically blood pressure. Our bodies respond to stress with a surge of hormones, including cortisol and adrenaline, which temporarily increase blood pressure.

This temporary rise in blood pressure is natural and not typically a concern. However, continuous exposure to stress, and hence a persistently elevated level of these hormones, can lead to sustained high blood pressure—a risk factor for heart disease.

Meditation enters the scene as a powerful stress-busting tool that can mitigate this risk. By invoking a state of deep relaxation, meditation encourages the body to lower the production of stress hormones, reducing their impact on the cardiovascular system. This state of tranquility not only tempers the immediate stress response but also contributes to reducing baseline blood pressure levels over time.

Moreover, scientific investigations have uncovered substantial evidence supporting the positive influence of consistent meditation on blood pressure. In particular, transcendental meditation, a specialized variant of the practice, has been linked with appreciable decreases in both upper (systolic) and lower (diastolic) blood pressure readings. It involves the silent repetition of a personal mantra, which is a word or phrase in a specific manner. The objective is to induce a state of relaxed awareness that facilitates the release of stress and fatigue from the mind and body.

In a study conducted by Joanne Kraenzle Schneider, Chuntana Reangsing, and Danny G. Willis (2022), the impact of this particular form of meditation on blood pressure was found. Their findings indicated that TM could lead to a modest decrease in blood pressure, although this effect tends to diminish after approximately three months. Additionally, they observed that older adults above the age of 65 appeared to derive greater benefits compared to younger adults.

However, it is important to note that the researchers were cautious in interpreting these findings. They emphasized that Transcendental Meditation should be viewed as one aspect of a heart-healthy lifestyle rather than a standalone solution for high blood pressure.

This perspective aligns with the broader philosophy of complementary and alternative medicine, which promotes holistic and comprehensive approaches to health and well-being. Therefore, while TM may not produce significant and long-lasting reductions in blood pressure on its own, it can still contribute to an overall strategy for managing blood pressure and promoting heart health, particularly when combined with other lifestyle adjustments such as dietary changes, exercise, and stress management.

Another study conducted by James W. Anderson, Chunxu Liu, and Richard J Kryscio delves deeper into the impact of Transcendental Meditation on blood pressure. The findings suggest that practicing Transcendental Meditation can potentially lead to clinically significant changes, with systolic blood pressure decreasing by approximately 4.7 mm Hg and diastolic blood pressure decreasing by 3.2 mm Hg.

Although these reductions may appear modest, they can hold great clinical importance. Even a slight decrease in blood pressure can substantially reduce the risk of heart disease and stroke. Therefore, these findings highlight the potential value of Transcendental Meditation as part of a comprehensive approach to managing high blood pressure.

In addition to its effects on blood pressure, the researchers also observed a range of other health benefits associated with regular Transcendental Meditation practice. These benefits encompass anxiety reduction, improved sleep quality, and enhanced overall well-being.

Consequently, this study not only reinforces the potential of Transcendental Meditation as a tool for blood pressure management but also emphasizes that the advantages of such practices extend beyond physical health. The promotion of mental and emotional well-being, better sleep, and reduced anxiety are all integral aspects of a holistic approach to health. This further underscores the value of incorporating techniques like Transcendental Meditation into a comprehensive health and wellness strategy.

How to Meditate

Meditation can seem like an intricate and daunting practice, but its core concept is straightforward—stilling the mind to bring about a sense of inner peace and self-awareness. Here's a simplified step-by-step guide to meditation:

1. **Find a Peaceful Location**: Choose a serene spot where you won't be disturbed during your meditation session. It could be a quiet room in

your house, a tranquil garden, or even a quiet park.

2. **Choose a Comfortable Position**: Sit comfortably. You can opt to sit on a chair, cross-legged on the floor, or even lie down if that's more comfortable for you. The goal is to find a position where you can remain relaxed yet attentive.

3. **Focus Your Attention**: Close your eyes and start focusing on your breath. Observe the sensation of your breath as it flows in and out. Try not to control your breath but rather just observe its natural rhythm.

4. **Be Mindful:** Your mind will inevitably wander, and that's okay. Whenever you realize that your thoughts have drifted, gently redirect your focus back to your breath without judging yourself.

5. **Start Small and Gradually Increase Duration**: Start by meditating for just a few minutes a day, then gradually increase your practice time as you feel comfortable. Even a few minutes of meditation can make a difference.

6. **Practice Regularly**: Consistency is key in meditation. Make it a part of your daily routine to get the most benefit out of the practice.

Remember, meditation is not about attaining perfection but rather about improving awareness and acceptance. It's perfectly normal to have days when meditation feels more challenging. What matters most is that you persist and continue the practice.

Also, while meditation is a powerful tool in managing stress and improving blood pressure, it should not be considered a standalone treatment for high blood pressure. It is best utilized as a complementary approach alongside traditional blood pressure management strategies. As always, any changes to your health regimen should be discussed with a healthcare professional.

Yoga

Yoga offers a holistic approach to managing blood pressure by addressing both physical and mental well-being. Through regular practice, yoga has been shown to effectively reduce stress levels, which can contribute to high blood pressure. By engaging in various yoga techniques, individuals can experience a decrease in stress hormones and a promotion of relaxation, ultimately leading to lower blood pressure levels.

In addition to stress reduction, yoga can enhance overall fitness and cardiovascular health. Certain forms of yoga, such as Vinyasa or Power Yoga, involve dynamic movements and increased physical exertion, which can improve cardiovascular endurance. This aspect of yoga is particularly advantageous for individuals with high blood pressure, as it helps to strengthen the heart and improve its efficiency.

A comprehensive study published in Mayo Clinic Proceedings in 2019 further supports the positive effects of yoga on blood pressure. The research focused on overweight, middle-aged adults with high blood pressure who practiced yoga for about an hour five times a week over a period of 13 weeks. The study revealed significant reductions in blood pressure among the participants. Furthermore, when the yoga sessions incorporated specific breathing techniques and meditation, the improvements in blood pressure were even more pronounced.

These findings emphasize the potential of yoga as a valuable tool in blood pressure management. By integrating physical postures, breathing exercises, and meditation, yoga provides a comprehensive approach to promoting cardiovascular health and reducing stress. As with any exercise or therapeutic practice, it's advisable to consult with a healthcare professional before starting a yoga routine, especially for individuals with pre-existing medical conditions.

Yoga Poses – Lower Blood Pressure

Incorporating yoga into your lifestyle can be a powerful tool in managing and reducing high blood pressure. Yoga combines physical postures, controlled breathing, and mindfulness to promote overall health and well-being.

Along with its numerous benefits for the body and mind, yoga has been shown to positively affect blood pressure levels. By practicing specific yoga poses that target relaxation, stress reduction, and circulation you can support your cardiovascular health and work toward maintaining a healthy blood pressure range.

In this section, I will take you through six yoga poses that are particularly beneficial for reducing high blood pressure. By integrating these poses into your regular practice, you can harness the therapeutic benefits of yoga and embark on a journey toward better heart health and overall well-being.

1. Balasana (Child's Pose): Balasana, or Child's Pose, is a gentle and relaxing yoga posture that can help reduce high blood pressure. Start kneeling on the mat with your toes touching and knees slightly apart. Slowly lower your hips toward your heels and rest your forehead on the mat. Extend your arms alongside your body or place them gently on the mat above your head. Take slow, deep breaths, allowing your body to relax and release tension. Balasana promotes a sense of calmness and relaxation, helping to reduce stress and lower blood pressure.

2. Paschimottanasana (Seated Forward Bend): Paschimottanasana, or Seated Forward Bend, is a seated yoga pose that stretches the entire back of the body, promoting relaxation and relieving tension. Sit on the mat with your legs extended in front of you. Slowly bend forward from the hips, reaching your hands toward your feet or resting them on your shins or thighs. Keep your spine long and your gaze forward. Breathe deeply and relax into the pose, allowing your body to gently release tension. Paschimottanasana helps to calm the mind, reduce stress, and regulate blood pressure.

3. Baddha Konasana (Bound Angle Pose): Baddha Konasana, or Bound Angle Pose, is a seated posture that opens the hips and promotes relaxation. Sit on the mat with your legs bent and the soles of your feet touching each other. Hold your feet or ankles with your hands and gently press your knees toward the floor. Sit tall and lengthen your spine, allowing your hips to open and your inner thighs to stretch. Take slow, deep breaths, focusing on relaxing your body and mind. Baddha Konasana helps relieve anxiety, improve circulation, and support healthy blood pressure.

4. Janu Sirsasana (Head-to-Knee Pose): Janu Sirsasana, or Head-to-Knee Pose, is a seated forward bend that stretches the hamstrings and calms the nervous system. Sit on the mat with one leg extended and the sole of the other foot against your inner thigh. Slowly fold forward, reaching toward your extended leg with your hands. Keep your spine long and breathe deeply as you relax into the pose. Janu Sirsasana helps to release tension, reduce stress, and promote healthy blood pressure levels.

5. Virasana (Hero Pose) with extended exhale breathing: Virasana, or Hero Pose, is a kneeling posture that opens the chest, promotes relaxation, and supports healthy blood pressure. Start by kneeling on the mat with your knees together and your feet slightly apart. Sit back on your heels and lengthen your spine. Place your hands on your thighs or rest them on your knees. Take slow, deep breaths, and as you exhale, extend the length of your breath, allowing your exhalations to be longer than your inhalations. Virasana, with extended exhale breathing, helps to activate the parasympathetic nervous system, reduce stress, and regulate blood pressure.

6. Savasana (Corpse Pose): Savasana, or Corpse Pose, is a deeply relaxing and restorative posture that allows the body and mind to fully relax. Lie on your back with your legs extended and your arms resting alongside your body, palms facing up. Close your eyes and focus on your breath, allowing it to flow naturally and deeply. Release any tension in your body and surrender to a state of complete relaxation. Savasana helps to reduce stress, lower blood pressure, and promote overall well-being. It allows for deep rest and rejuvenation, supporting the body's natural healing processes.

VITAMINS

Vitamins are essential organic compounds that are required in small amounts for the body's normal functioning. They play a crucial role in various physiological processes, such as metabolism, growth, and maintenance of overall health. Vitamins are classified into two main types: fat-soluble and water-soluble.

Fat-soluble vitamins, as the name suggests, dissolve and are stored in the body's fatty tissues. These include vitamins A, D, E, and K. Fat-soluble vitamins are absorbed through the intestines and dietary fats and stored in the liver and fatty tissues for future use. Because they can be stored, excess consumption of fat-soluble vitamins can potentially lead to toxicity.

On the other hand, water-soluble vitamins, including vitamin C and the B-complex vitamins (such as B1, B2, B3, B5, B6, B7, B9, and B12) are not stored in the body to a significant extent. They dissolve in water and are easily absorbed into the bloodstream. Water-soluble vitamins are not stored in large quantities, and any excess amounts are excreted through urine. Therefore, regular intake of water-soluble vitamins is important to meet the body's requirements.

Both types of vitamins are essential for maintaining optimal health, but it's important to note that the body's requirements for each vitamin may vary. A balanced diet that includes a variety of foods can provide an adequate intake of vitamins. However, in certain cases, such as pregnancy, illness, or specific dietary restrictions, supplementation may be recommended under the guidance of a healthcare professional to ensure sufficient vitamin intake.

MINERALS

Minerals are vital micronutrients that our bodies require in relatively small amounts to support various physiological functions. They are essential for maintaining overall health and well-being. Let's explore some of the different types of minerals and their roles in the body, particularly their importance for individuals with high blood pressure:

1. **Calcium**: Calcium is well known for its role in promoting strong bones and teeth. It also plays a crucial role in regulating blood pressure by assisting in constricting and relaxing blood vessels.
2. **Magnesium:** Magnesium is involved in over 300 biochemical reactions in the body. It helps relax blood vessels, thereby contributing to the maintenance of healthy blood pressure levels.
3. **Potassium:** Potassium is an electrolyte that helps balance the fluids and minerals in the body. It plays a vital role in regulating blood pressure by counteracting the effects of sodium and supporting healthy heart function.
4. **Sodium:** While excessive sodium intake can contribute to high blood pressure, a moderate amount of sodium is necessary for maintaining fluid balance and supporting proper nerve and muscle function.
5. **Zinc:** Zinc is involved in numerous enzymatic reactions and plays a crucial role in immune function, wound healing, and cell division. It indirectly contributes to blood pressure

regulation by supporting overall cardiovascular health.

6. **Iron:** Iron is essential for the production of red blood cells, which transport oxygen throughout the body. Adequate iron levels are crucial for maintaining optimal blood pressure and preventing conditions associated with iron deficiency.

For individuals with high blood pressure, maintaining appropriate mineral levels is important. A balanced diet that includes a variety of nutrient-rich foods such as fruits, vegetables, whole grains, lean proteins, and low-fat dairy products can provide an adequate intake of minerals.

In this regard, it is important to remember that certain medical conditions or medications may affect mineral levels, so consulting with a healthcare professional or registered dietitian is recommended to tailor a dietary plan that suits individual needs. By incorporating a variety of mineral-rich foods into their diet, blood pressure patients can support their overall health and contribute to the management of their condition.

FOOD OR SUPPLEMENTS

When it comes to obtaining vitamins and minerals, it is generally recommended to prioritize food as the primary source. Whole foods provide a wide array of essential nutrients, along with other beneficial compounds such as fiber and antioxidants.

The body is designed to absorb and utilize vitamins and minerals more efficiently from food sources, as they come packaged with other synergistic components that work together for optimal absorption and utilization. While supplements can be helpful in certain situations, such as addressing specific deficiencies or supporting certain health conditions, they should not replace a well-balanced diet.

Whole foods offer the added advantage of providing a diverse range of nutrients and phytochemicals that support overall health and well-being. Therefore, focusing on a nutrient-rich diet, including a variety of fruits, vegetables, whole grains, lean proteins, and healthy fats, is the best approach to meet the body's vitamin and mineral needs.

In most cases, the absorption of vitamins and minerals from natural food sources tends to be more efficient compared to their synthetic counterparts in supplement form.

Choosing a well-rounded, nutrient-dense diet over relying solely on supplements provides a multitude of benefits, as whole foods offer a wide spectrum of nutrients, fiber, and antioxidants that contribute to overall health and well-being. However, it's important to acknowledge that relying solely on food for all necessary vitamins and minerals can pose challenges.

Access to a diverse range of nutrient-rich foods may be limited for some individuals due to various factors such as geographical location, economic constraints, or personal dietary restrictions. Additionally, factors like soil quality, food processing, and cooking methods can affect the nutrient content of foods, making it challenging to guarantee sufficient intake through diet alone.

In such cases, supplements can be a helpful tool to fill potential nutritional gaps and address specific deficiencies. They can provide concentrated doses of certain vitamins and minerals, especially when prescribed by healthcare professionals. It is crucial, though, to approach supplements as complementary to a healthy diet rather than a substitute.

Relying solely on supplements while neglecting a balanced eating pattern can lead to a lack of other essential nutrients and the associated benefits they provide. Striking a balance between obtaining nutrients from whole foods and considering targeted supplementation when necessary can help ensure optimal nutrient intake.

DIETARY SUPPLEMENTS

Dietary supplements are products intended to supplement one's diet and provide additional nutrients, such as vitamins, minerals, herbs, or other botanicals, amino acids, or enzymes. They come in various forms, including capsules, tablets, powders, liquids, or even energy bars.

The benefits of dietary supplements lie in their ability to fill potential nutritional gaps and support overall health and well-being. They can be particularly beneficial for individuals with specific dietary restrictions, limited access to nutrient-rich foods, or increased nutrient needs due to certain life stages or health conditions.

Supplements can help bridge nutritional deficiencies and ensure adequate intake of essential vitamins, minerals, and other vital nutrients. It's also important to keep in mind that prior to incorporating any dietary supplements into your routine, it is crucial to consult with your doctor to verify that they will not interfere with any medications you are currently taking or result in any undesirable consequences.

Even though natural supplements may be considered safe, it is essential to recognize that they can still induce side effects, particularly when consumed in excessive quantities or for prolonged durations. Additionally, it is advisable to undergo laboratory tests and undergo a micronutrient assessment to gain insights into your current nutrient levels before initiating any supplement plan.

MICRONUTRIENT TESTS

A micronutrient test is a specialized assessment that offers valuable information regarding the presence of any nutrient deficiencies or imbalances within your body. By analyzing your blood or other bodily samples, this test can identify specific micronutrient levels and provide insights into your individual nutritional needs.

This knowledge can be instrumental in determining which dietary supplements may be most beneficial for addressing any deficiencies or imbalances. To ensure an accurate interpretation of the results and appropriate supplementation, it is recommended to consult with your healthcare provider. They can guide you in selecting the most suitable micronutrient test for your circumstances and help you understand the significance of the findings.

Understanding your micronutrient status through testing allows you and your healthcare provider to develop a more targeted approach to your nutritional supplementation. By identifying the nutrients that may be lacking or imbalanced, you can choose the appropriate dietary supplements to address those specific needs.

It's important to remember that dietary supplements are designed to complement a healthy and balanced diet, not to serve as a substitute for it. Emphasizing whole foods as the primary source of nutrients is essential for overall well-being. Supplements should be used judiciously and, only when necessary, to support and enhance your overall health and wellness journey.

SUPPLEMENTS FOR YOU

Various supplements have a crucial role in meeting the dietary requirements of individuals with hypertension. They serve as a valuable source of extra nutrients that may be deficient in their regular diet, aiding in the promotion of overall well-being and the regulation of blood pressure.

Specific supplements like magnesium, potassium, and CoQ10 have been linked to the reduction of blood pressure levels. Additionally, the inclusion of omega-3 fatty acids from fish oil supplements can contribute to cardiovascular health. These supplements offer an effective means of supplementing one's diet to address nutritional gaps and support the management of blood pressure.

Some of the most important supplements include the following:

Magnesium: Magnesium is crucial for regulating blood pressure and muscle function. Optimal magnesium levels have been linked to lower blood pressure.

Vitamin D: Insufficient vitamin D has been associated with hypertension. Taking vitamin D supplements may help maintain healthy blood pressure.

B vitamins: B vitamins, such as folate, vitamin B6, and vitamin B12, play a role in cardiovascular health and maintaining optimal blood pressure.

Potassium: Essential for balancing sodium levels, potassium helps support healthy blood pressure. Adequate intake through supplements or potassium-rich foods is beneficial.

CoQ10: Coenzyme Q10 (CoQ10) is an antioxidant involved in cellular energy production. Studies suggest that CoQ10 supplementation may contribute to lower blood pressure.

L-arginine: L-arginine, an amino acid, promotes the production of nitric oxide, which aids in blood vessel relaxation and improves blood flow, potentially benefiting blood pressure.

Vitamin C: As an antioxidant, vitamin C may enhance blood vessel function and promote healthy blood pressure levels.

Beetroot: Rich in nitrates, beetroot can be converted to nitric oxide, supporting blood vessel dilation, and potentially reducing blood pressure.

Garlic: Garlic has long been recognized for its cardiovascular benefits, including maintaining healthy blood pressure.

Fish oil: Omega-3 fatty acids in fish oil offer cardiovascular advantages, including support for healthy blood pressure.

Probiotics: Select probiotic strains may contribute to cardiovascular health, including the maintenance of healthy blood pressure levels.

Melatonin: Melatonin, a hormone involved in sleep-wake cycles, may modestly impact blood pressure regulation.

Green tea: Green tea contains catechins, compounds with antioxidants and blood pressure-lowering properties.

Ginger: Ginger has been studied for potential cardio-vascular benefits, including its impact on healthy blood pressure levels.

Vitamin K2: Vitamin K2 aids in calcium metabolism and vascular health, potentially influencing blood pressure regulation.

Caution: When contemplating the utilization of vitamins for managing blood pressure, it is crucial to approach it with caution and take necessary precautions. The foremost step is to seek advice from your healthcare professional before initiating any new supplements.

If you are taking blood thinners, avoid the consumption of Vitamin K2. Blood thinners work by inhibiting the formation of blood clotting factors that depend on vitamin K. Taking vitamin K can interfere with the intended effects of blood thinners, counteracting their effectiveness. It is important to consult with your healthcare provider or pharmacist to understand potential interactions and to ensure the safe and appropriate use of Vitamin K2 or any other supplements while on blood thinners.

COMMIT TO THE JOURNEY

If lifestyle modifications alone do not yield the desired results in lowering blood pressure within a span of six months, a recent scientific statement by the American Heart Association proposes maintaining those healthy habits while also contemplating the inclusion of blood pressure-lowering medications.

The journey of managing hypertension can be a lengthy endeavor, but the rewards that come with it are unquestionably worthwhile. Lowering blood pressure requires a holistic approach, encompassing medications, lifestyle modifications, and complementary or alternative therapies.

It's important to recognize that the desired outcomes may not manifest instantly; rather, it may take several weeks or even months to witness the full effects of these interventions. Despite the challenges that may arise during this process, maintaining unwavering commitment and adhering to your personalized plan is fundamental to achieving success.

Perseverance and resilience play vital roles, as consistency is the key to attaining long-lasting results. Even

214 | DR. ASHLEY SULLIVAN, PHARMD, RPH, MBA

when progress appears gradual, faithfully integrating the recommended changes into your daily routine will contribute to a healthier and more enriching life.

It's crucial to remain mindful of the fact that the path to improved blood pressure management is an ongoing journey that demands patience and unwavering dedication. In the upcoming chapter, we will delve into understanding the consequences of not checking high blood pressure.

9

THE HIDDEN DANGERS

Various risks and complications exist with uncontrolled hypertension. In fact, a fundamental challenge in the field of medicine lies in the realm of uncertainty, which permeates the experiences of patients, doctors, and society at large. In *Complications: A Surgeon's Notes on an Imperfect Science* Atul Gawande remarkably stated that despite the progress we have made in understanding human health, diseases, and their treatments, the pervasive nature of uncertainty remains elusive.

As a patient, navigating through this uncertainty can be emotionally distressing, while doctors face the constant struggle of grappling with the vast expanse of the unknown. It becomes evident that the essence of medical care resides not solely in what is known but rather in acknowledging and addressing what remains uncertain. Uncertainty forms the bedrock of medicine, and the ability to navigate it wisely becomes a defining factor in both the patient's and doctor's journey.

The field of medicine encompasses more than just precise calculations and definitive solutions. Even with the most advanced treatments available, there are inherent uncertainties and unknown factors that permeate the management of health conditions.

However, in the case of high blood pressure, the risks and potential complications associated with uncontrolled hypertension are widely acknowledged and substantial. Despite some degree of uncertainty regarding the ideal treatment approach, the dangers posed by unmanaged high blood pressure are evident.

They range from detrimental effects on vital organs like the heart, brain, and kidneys to an increased susceptibility to life-threatening events such as stroke. By prioritizing blood pressure management and maintaining close collaboration with healthcare professionals, individuals can effectively minimize the risks and uncertainties.

Gaining an understanding of these risks and complications is paramount to taking proactive measures in blood pressure management and ensuring optimal long-term health. Moreover, when it comes to high blood pressure, risks and complications are interconnected concepts, each with its own distinct meaning.

- Risks pertain to factors or conditions that heighten the probability of a particular event occurring.
- Complications, on the other hand, encompass the adverse health outcomes that can arise as a consequence of a given condition.

Furthermore, risks encompass various factors that can increase the likelihood of developing the condition or experiencing related health issues. These factors may include family history, certain lifestyle choices, or underlying medical conditions.

On the other hand, complications associated with high blood pressure involve the negative health consequences that can manifest when the condition is left uncontrolled. These complications can range from cardiovascular problems, such as heart attack or stroke, to damage to organs like the kidneys or brain.

RISKS AND COMPLICATIONS OF UNCONTROLLED HYPERTENSION

When it comes to high blood pressure, several risks and complications can make matters worse. In this section, we'll be walking through some of the major ones.

Damaged and narrowed arteries

Increased blood pressure can result in harm to the inner lining of arteries. This damage can worsen when fats from the diet accumulate in the bloodstream. The combined effect of arterial damage and fat buildup can diminish the flexibility of artery walls, impeding the smooth flow of blood throughout the body. This reduced blood flow over an extended period can give rise to various complications, such as heart disease, stroke, and damage to other organs and tissues in the body.

Aneurysm

Consistently elevated blood pressure increases the pressure on weakened areas of the arteries. This prolonged pressure can cause further weakening of the arterial wall, potentially leading to an aneurysm. As the artery endures heightened stress, the weakened segment may enlarge and possibly rupture, resulting in severe internal bleeding that poses a life-threatening risk.

While not all aneurysms are directly caused by high blood pressure, hypertension can contribute to their formation and elevate the risk of complications. Maintaining blood pressure within a healthy range is crucial to reduce the chances of aneurysm development and rupture.

Through effective blood pressure management involving lifestyle adjustments, prescribed medications, and regular monitoring, individuals can significantly decrease the likelihood of developing an aneurysm. Collaborating closely with healthcare professionals enables the creation of a comprehensive plan encompassing routine blood pressure checks, the adoption of healthy eating habits, regular exercise, stress reduction techniques, and adherence to prescribed medications.

Always remember that preventing aneurysms begins with maintaining a healthy blood pressure level. By taking proactive measures to manage hypertension, you can safeguard those blood vessels and diminish the risks associated with aneurysm formation.

Damage to the heart

Elevated blood pressure disrupts the functioning of the endothelial system, posing a considerable risk for the development of atherosclerotic disease, coronary artery disease, and peripheral arterial disease (Tackling & Borhade, 2022). Hypertension can cause damage to the arteries and result in their narrowing, impeding the flow of blood to the heart.

This reduction in blood flow can manifest as chest pain, irregular heart rhythms, and, in severe cases, heart attacks. When left uncontrolled, high blood pressure can lead to the narrowing and impairment of arteries, depriving the heart of sufficient blood supply.

Enlarged left ventricle

Elevated blood pressure forces the heart to exert more effort in pumping blood across the body. This added strain can result in the thickening of the left ventricle of the heart, heightening the chances of heart attack, heart failure, and sudden cardiac death.

When high blood pressure remains uncontrolled, the left ventricle of the heart may thicken, compromising its ability to function effectively. This condition, referred to as left ventricular hypertrophy, increases the susceptibility to severe heart complications, including heart attacks and heart failure.

Heart failure

As time passes, elevated blood pressure can exert pressure on the heart, leading to strain. This strain can result in the weakening of the heart muscle and a decline in its efficiency. If the strain persists over an extended period, it can eventually lead to heart failure, where the heart's ability to pump blood adequately becomes compromised.

Damage to the brain

Transient Ischemic Attack (TIA)

A transient ischemic attack (TIA) is considered a mild form of stroke. It occurs when there is a temporary blockage or reduction in blood flow to a specific area of the brain, usually caused by a blood clot. Unlike a stroke, the symptoms of a TIA are similar but brief and do not result in lasting damage.

The blockage in a blood vessel supplying the brain can occur due to damage caused by high blood pressure or high cholesterol. Additionally, a blood clot from another location, such as the heart or neck blood vessels, can also travel to the brain and cause a TIA.

Often referred to as a ministroke, a TIA serves as a warning sign that a more severe stroke may occur in the future. It is crucial to address high blood pressure as it can contribute to the formation of hardened arteries or blood clots, increasing the risk of experiencing a TIA.

Stroke

Insufficient oxygen and nutrients reaching the brain can result in a stroke as the cells in the brain start to perish. High blood pressure can be detrimental to blood vessels in the brain, causing them to narrow, rupture, or leak, thereby increasing the likelihood of a stroke.

Furthermore, hypertension raises the risk of blood clots forming within the arteries that supply the brain, obstructing the flow of blood and potentially leading to a stroke. By damaging blood vessels and promoting clot formation, high blood pressure poses a significant threat to the occurrence of a stroke.

Dementia

Vascular dementia, a specific form of dementia, can manifest when the arteries supplying blood to the brain undergo narrowing or blockage. This leads to the restriction of blood flow and causes harm to brain cells.

Additionally, a stroke that disrupts blood flow to the brain can contribute to the development of vascular dementia, as it inflicts considerable damage and loss of brain cells, consequently impairing cognitive abilities and memory. In both cases, the compromised blood flow and subsequent damage to brain cells are key factors in the onset of vascular dementia—highlighting the critical importance of maintaining healthy blood circulation to preserve cognitive function.

Mild Cognitive Impairment

Mild cognitive impairment represents a transitional stage between typical age-related changes in cognition and more severe forms of dementia, characterized by noticeable alterations in memory and comprehension (NHS, 2019). Emerging evidence indicates that elevated blood pressure may play a role in the onset of mild cognitive impairment.

Research suggests that high blood pressure could be a contributing factor in the development of these cognitive changes, highlighting the potential link between hypertension and the early stages of cognitive decline.

Understanding the impact of blood pressure on cognitive health is crucial in identifying strategies to mitigate the risk and promote optimal brain function.

Damage to the kidneys

Kidney scarring (glomerulosclerosis)

High blood pressure can also impact the kidneys. A common condition that can develop is known as "Glomerulosclerosis." In this condition, tiny blood vessels within the kidneys undergo scarring.

As a result, the kidneys lose their ability to efficiently filter waste and fluid from the blood. The progression of glomerulosclerosis can ultimately lead to kidney failure, a critical and potentially life-threatening condition.

When the kidneys fail, they are unable to adequately perform their vital functions of removing waste and excess fluid from the body. Recognizing the implications of glomerulosclerosis is crucial as it highlights the significance of preserving kidney health and seeking appropriate medical intervention to prevent or manage kidney failure.

Kidney failure

High blood pressure stands as a primary contributor to the development of kidney failure. This arises from the potential damage inflicted upon the blood vessels responsible for supplying the kidneys, impeding their proper functioning.

When the kidneys are unable to efficiently filter waste and excess fluid from the blood, the accumulation of harmful levels within the body can ensue, leading to severe complications and, in some cases, kidney failure. To address kidney failure resulting from uncontrolled hypertension, treatment options such as dialysis or kidney transplantation may be necessary.

However, individuals can actively reduce their risk of kidney failure by effectively managing their blood pressure and collaborating with healthcare professionals to prevent and control kidney disease. Taking proactive steps in these regards significantly contributes to preserving kidney health and overall well-being.

Damage to the eyes

Retinopathy refers to the impairment of blood vessels in the retina caused by uncontrolled hypertension. This condition can give rise to various vision issues, including blurred vision and, in severe cases, complete vision loss.

Moreover, the damage inflicted upon the retinal blood vessels can result in bleeding within the eye, which presents a significant and potentially serious complication. Individuals with both high blood pressure and diabetes face an elevated risk of developing retinopathy, as these conditions collectively contribute to the deterioration of blood vessels in the eye. Thus, it is crucial to manage blood pressure levels effectively and address related conditions to minimize the risk of retinopathy and safeguard visual health.

Fluid buildup under the retina (Choroidopathy)

Choroidopathy is a condition that affects the blood vessels in the eye and can have detrimental effects on vision. It can manifest as distorted or blurry vision, and in more severe cases, it may result in scarring that can permanently impair vision.

The damage caused by choroidopathy can lead to various vision problems, including the distortion of images, making it difficult for individuals to see clearly. Consequently, managing choroidopathy is crucial to preserve visual acuity and minimize the impact on daily activities. Regular eye examinations and appropriate treatment can help mitigate the effects of choroidopathy and maintain optimal vision.

Nerve damage (Optic Neuropathy)

Impaired blood flow can adversely affect the optic nerve, leading to vision loss or intraocular bleeding.

Blockage of blood flow can result in damage to the optic nerve, causing the accumulation of blood within the eye or even partial or complete loss of vision.

When the optic nerve is compromised due to inadequate blood supply, it hampers the transmission of visual signals to the brain, leading to visual disturbances. It is important to address the obstruction of blood flow promptly to minimize the risk of optic nerve damage and preserve visual function. Seeking medical attention and adopting appropriate interventions can help mitigate the potential consequences of vision.

Sexual Dysfunction

In men aged 50 and above, it is common to encounter erectile dysfunction, a condition characterized by the inability to achieve or sustain an erection. However, men with high blood pressure face an even higher likelihood of experiencing erectile dysfunction, as hypertension can restrict the blood flow to the penis.

Similarly, women with high blood pressure may also encounter challenges in sexual functioning. High blood pressure can lead to diminished blood flow to the vagina, resulting in decreased sexual desire, difficulty getting aroused, vaginal dryness, and difficulties in achieving orgasm. These effects on sexual health emphasize the importance of managing blood pressure to promote a satisfying and fulfilling sexual experience for both men and women.

PREVENTING RISKS AND COMPLICATIONS

To prevent the risks and complications associated with uncontrolled high blood pressure, a comprehensive approach that combines lifestyle modifications and medication is often necessary. Here are some strategies that can help you in dealing with these complications:

- Regularly monitor your blood pressure and collaborate with your healthcare provider to develop a personalized management plan.
- Implement lifestyle changes that support healthy blood pressure levels, such as adopting a heart-healthy diet, engaging in regular physical activity, managing stress effectively, and quitting smoking.
- Adhere to prescribed medications as directed by your doctor and be mindful of any potential side effects or interactions with other medications, supplements, or food.
- Manage other underlying health conditions that can contribute to high blood pressure or

increase your risk of complications, such as diabetes or high cholesterol.

- Pay attention to any symptoms or warning signs of a complication, such as chest pain, shortness of breath, severe headache, or changes in vision, and seek prompt medical attention if they arise.
- By taking a proactive approach to managing your blood pressure, you can significantly reduce the risk of complications and enhance your overall health and well-being.

Remember, effective blood pressure management requires a comprehensive and ongoing effort involving both self-care measures and regular communication with your healthcare provider. By prioritizing your health and implementing these preventive measures, you can take control of your blood pressure and promote a healthier future.

Now, transitioning from the discussion on the potential risks and complications associated with uncontrolled high blood pressure, let's shift our focus to a more proactive approach. One effective way to take charge of your health and reduce the risk of complications is by regularly monitoring your blood pressure.

By actively tracking your blood pressure levels, you empower yourself to make informed decisions and take necessary steps toward maintaining a healthier blood pressure range. This proactive approach enables you to stay vigilant, identify any fluctuations, and work toward achieving optimal blood pressure levels for better overall health and a reduced risk of complications. In the next chapter, we'll take a look at how you can stay in control of your health.

10

STAY ON TOP OF YOUR HEALTH

" *"In the long run, we shape our lives and ourselves. The process never ends until we die. And the choices we make are ultimately our own responsibility."*

— ELEANOR ROOSEVELT

These profound words of Eleanor Roosevelt serve as a powerful reminder that our lives are a culmination of the choices we make. When it comes to managing high blood pressure, this truth resonates deeply. By taking an active role in our own health journey, we hold the key to influencing our well-being and paving the path toward a healthier future.

In this chapter, I will take you through the significance of self-monitoring blood pressure and its capacity to empower us in safeguarding our cardiovascular health. We will uncover the reasons why tracking our blood pressure readings goes beyond being merely beneficial —it becomes an indispensable tool in effectively managing hypertension.

Imagine the ability to monitor your blood pressure at your convenience, anytime and anywhere, liberating you from relying solely on sporadic visits to the doctor's office. By creating a personalized logbook to record your readings, you open the door to valuable insights into your blood pressure patterns, enabling you to identify triggers and make well-informed decisions regarding your lifestyle and treatment plan.

Throughout the pages ahead, I will guide you in establishing your blood pressure logbook, providing practical tips and strategies to make the process seamless and enjoyable. I will discuss various methods of measuring blood pressure, emphasizing the significance of accurate readings, and address common challenges you may encounter on this empowering journey.

Moreover, together, we will explore the numerous benefits of self-monitoring, including heightened awareness of your blood pressure fluctuations, improved communication with your healthcare provider, and the ability to detect concerning trends at their earliest stages. Armed with this knowledge, you become an active participant in your own healthcare, working hand in hand with your medical team to achieve optimal blood pressure control.

It is crucial to remember that taking charge of your blood pressure is not a fleeting commitment but a life-long responsibility. It entails embracing your role in caring for your well-being and consciously making choices that positively impact your health. Together, let us embark on this voyage of self-monitoring and empowerment, unlocking the boundless potential to shape a future marked by improved health and unbridled happiness.

SELF-MONITORING YOUR BLOOD PRESSURE

Self-monitoring blood pressure is a critical aspect of managing hypertension and promoting overall cardio-vascular health. This proactive approach empowers you to take control of your well-being, make informed deci-sions, and work collaboratively with healthcare profes-sionals to achieve optimal blood pressure control.

Moreover, regularly monitoring your blood pressure at home enables you to develop a deeper comprehension of your condition and make informed choices regarding treatment and lifestyle adjustments. Some reasons why self-monitoring blood pressure is so important are:

1. Enhanced Awareness: Self-monitoring blood pressure fosters a deeper comprehension of the factors influencing blood pressure levels. Through regular tracking of readings, individuals develop a heightened awareness of how lifestyle choices, stress, and various activities impact their blood pressure. This increased awareness empowers them to make informed decisions about their daily routines and make necessary adjustments to promote better control of their blood pressure.

2. Improved Blood Pressure Management: Self-monitoring empowers individuals to actively take charge of their blood pressure on a daily basis. By consistently tracking readings, individuals can identify patterns and triggers that contribute to elevated blood pressure. Armed with this knowledge, they can make lifestyle modifications, such as adopting a healthier diet, increasing physical activity, managing stress, and adhering to prescribed medications. These proactive measures lead to better control of blood pressure and its maintenance over time.

3. Early Detection of Changes: Self-monitoring enables the timely detection of any fluctuations or sustained elevations in blood pressure. This prompt identification allows individuals to seek medical attention and necessary interventions when needed. By detecting changes early on, potential complications can be prevented or minimized, resulting in improved overall health outcomes.

4. Improved Communication with Healthcare Providers: Self-monitored blood pressure readings serve as a valuable tool for effective communication with healthcare providers. By sharing accurate and consistent data, individuals can engage in meaningful discussions about their blood pressure management.

This collaborative approach fosters a partnership between individuals and their healthcare team, ensuring treatment plans are adjusted and optimized based on real-time information. It also enables healthcare providers to make well-informed decisions regarding medication adjustments, lifestyle modifications, and other interventions for achieving optimal blood pressure control.

By incorporating self-monitoring of blood pressure into daily routines, individuals can reap numerous benefits, including heightened awareness of blood pressure triggers, improved blood pressure management, early detection of changes, and enhanced communication with healthcare providers. Actively participating in monitoring and managing blood pressure empowers individuals to take an active role in their cardiovascular health, working toward maintaining optimal well-being.

Furthermore, healthcare professionals may face challenges in determining whether your blood pressure consistently remains high or if it is only elevated during medical appointments. Several factors can contribute to fluctuations in blood pressure during a clinic visit, such as the presence of white-coat syndrome and masked hypertension.

White-coat syndrome refers to a situation where a patient experiences a temporary rise in blood pressure, specifically when it is measured in a medical setting, while their blood pressure remains normal in other environments, like their home.

Conversely, masked hypertension occurs when a patient's blood pressure appears normal during office visits, but they experience elevated blood pressure readings at other times of the day or in different settings. In both cases, the reliability of blood pressure measurements taken solely at the doctor's office becomes questionable.

The signs and symptoms of white coat syndrome include blood pressure readings that are higher than usual when measured in a medical setting, while readings outside of that environment are normal. White coat syndrome is often triggered by anxiety or stress related to medical settings or healthcare professionals. The anticipation of having blood pressure taken in a clinical setting can temporarily elevate blood pressure levels.

The signs and symptoms of masked hypertension are blood pressure readings that are normal during medical visits but elevated at other times or in different settings. Masked hypertension can be influenced by factors such as stress, physical activity, or environmental conditions that differ from the clinic setting. Monitoring blood pressure in various situations is crucial to capture the true fluctuations in blood pressure levels.

It is also important to note that higher blood pressure readings during a medical visit potentially lead to misdiagnosis or an inaccurate assessment of hypertension. This can be because engaging in physical activity shortly before a doctor's appointment can temporarily raise blood pressure due to increased heart rate and exertion. As a result, blood pressure readings taken during the visit may be elevated even if the individual's blood pressure is typically within a normal range.

There can also be an increase in blood pressure readings during a medical consultation, potentially influenced by emotional or psychological stress related to discussing health concerns. This happens when individuals are anxious or stressed about their health condition or the potential outcomes of the discussion; their blood pressure may temporarily rise. Consequently, readings during the appointment may be higher than their baseline blood pressure in a relaxed state.

These phenomena highlight the importance of self-monitoring blood pressure at home, as it provides a more comprehensive and accurate picture of your blood pressure patterns throughout the day and in various settings. By incorporating home blood pressure monitoring into your routine, you can contribute valuable data that helps healthcare professionals make well-informed decisions regarding your diagnosis, treatment, and overall management of hypertension.

MONITORING YOUR BLOOD PRESSURE AT HOME

Monitoring your blood pressure at home offers a powerful and efficient method to stay proactive about your cardiovascular well-being (American Heart Association, 2017). Regularly tracking your blood pressure readings in the comfort of your own surroundings provides invaluable insights into your blood pressure patterns, enabling you to take the necessary steps for maintaining optimal levels.

How to Utilize a Home Blood Pressure Monitor: Utilizing a home blood pressure monitor is a simple process that seamlessly fits into your routine. Begin by selecting a reliable and accurate monitor that aligns with your requirements. Adhere to the manufacturer's instructions to set up the device correctly and acquaint yourself with its features.

Properly position the cuff on your upper arm, following the provided guidelines, ensuring a snug fit without excessive tightness. Sit in a calm and relaxed environment with back support and feet flat on the floor. Rest for a few minutes prior to taking a reading, refraining from talking or moving during the measurement. Follow the device's prompts to obtain an accurate reading, and record the results in your blood pressure logbook or smartphone app.

Understanding Your Numbers: Understanding the meaning behind your blood pressure numbers is crucial for effective monitoring. Blood pressure is represented by two values: systolic pressure (the top number) and diastolic pressure (the bottom number).

The American Heart Association defines normal blood pressure as below 120/80 mmHg. Readings between

120–129 (systolic) and below 80 (diastolic) indicate elevated blood pressure. Hypertension is categorized into two stages: stage 1 (130–139/80–89) and stage 2 (140 or higher/90 or higher). Familiarize yourself with these numbers and consult your healthcare provider for personalized guidance and target ranges based on your medical history and risk factors.

Responding to High Blood Pressure Readings: Obtaining a high blood pressure reading at home should not cause panic. Take a deep breath and remain composed, remembering that individual readings can fluctuate throughout the day due to various factors.

If consistently recording high readings, it is crucial to reach out to your healthcare provider to discuss the results and seek further evaluation. They can determine if lifestyle adjustments, medication modifications, or additional tests are necessary.

Selecting a Home Blood Pressure Monitor: Choosing the right home blood pressure monitor is essential for accurate and dependable readings. Consider factors such as cuff size, ease of use, display readability, and validated accuracy.

Seek monitors validated by reputable organizations like the Association for the Advancement of Medical Instrumentation (AAMI) or the British Hypertension

Society (BHS). Consult with your healthcare provider for recommendations regarding specific models or brands that suit your needs.

Left-Arm vs. Right-Arm Blood Pressure: When monitoring your blood pressure at home, establish consistency in arm selection. Both the left and right arms can provide accurate readings, but it is recommended to consistently use either arm for monitoring. This ensures measurement consistency and facilitates easier comparison of readings over time.

Monitoring your blood pressure at home places you in control of your health. By following proper techniques, comprehending your numbers, seeking professional guidance when required, and selecting a reliable monitor, you can effectively track your blood pressure and work toward maintaining optimal cardiovascular health.

KEEPING A BLOOD PRESSURE LOGBOOK

Keeping a blood pressure logbook is an invaluable tool for effectively managing your blood pressure and gaining deeper insights into your cardiovascular well-being. This logbook acts as a complete record of your blood pressure readings, enabling you to monitor trends, identify patterns, and make informed decisions concerning your lifestyle and treatment regimen. Here are the essential components of a blood pressure logbook:

1. Date and Time of Readings: Recording the date and time of each blood pressure reading is crucial for tracking your progress over time. This information allows you to observe any changes or trends that may occur throughout the day or over extended periods.

2. Systolic and Diastolic Blood Pressure Numbers: The logbook should include sections to record the systolic and diastolic blood pressure numbers for each reading. The systolic pressure represents the force exerted on artery walls when the heart contracts, while the diastolic pressure reflects the pressure when the heart is at rest between beats. Monitoring both values provides a comprehensive understanding of your blood pressure levels.

3. Heart Rate: In addition to blood pressure readings, monitoring your heart rate is valuable for assessing your cardiovascular health. Note your heart rate alongside each blood pressure reading to monitor any changes or irregularities.

4. Medications Taken: Allocate a section in the logbook to document the medications you have taken before each blood pressure reading. This information helps you evaluate the effectiveness of your medications and their impact on your blood pressure levels.

5. Notes on Symptoms or Lifestyle Changes: Develop a habit of jotting down any symptoms or lifestyle changes that may influence your blood pressure. For example, if you experience stress, engage in physical activity, consume caffeine, or make significant dietary changes, record these factors. These notes assist in identifying potential triggers or patterns that affect your blood pressure readings.

By consistently maintaining a blood pressure logbook, you possess a comprehensive record that enables you and your healthcare provider to review your progress, make informed adjustments to your treatment plan, and develop personalized strategies for effectively managing your blood pressure.

Tips for accuracy and consistency

1. Choose a Reliable Blood Pressure Monitor: Invest in a high-quality blood pressure monitor that has been validated and approved by reputable organizations like the Association for the Advancement of Medical Instrumentation (AAMI) or the British Hypertension Society (BHS). Regularly calibrate and maintain the monitor to ensure accurate readings.

244 | DR. ASHLEY SULLIVAN, PHARMD, RPH, MBA

2. Maintain a Consistent Measurement Schedule: Establish a fixed routine for measuring your blood pressure. Aim to take readings at the same time each day to minimize variations caused by daily fluctuations. Recommended times include mornings before taking medications and evenings before bedtime.

3. Use a Standardized Recording System: Keep a standardized record sheet or utilize a digital blood pressure tracking app. This promotes consistency in documenting your blood pressure readings, making it easier to identify trends and share the information with your healthcare provider. Include essential details such as date, time, blood pressure readings, heart rate, and any relevant notes.

4. Select a Quiet Environment for Measurements: Choose a calm and quiet location for taking blood pressure readings. Minimize distractions and external influences that could impact your blood pressure, such as noise or interruptions. Sit in a comfortable chair with proper back support and ensure your feet are flat on the floor, as this helps obtain accurate readings.

5. Record Each Reading Promptly: After measuring your blood pressure, immediately record the results in your log sheet or digital tracking app. This ensures precise and timely documentation, reducing the risk of errors or misinterpretation. Avoid delays in recording to maintain the accuracy of your log.

6. Share Your Log with Your Healthcare Provider: During check-ups or appointments, share your blood pressure log sheet or digital records with your healthcare provider. This enables them to review your progress, identify any concerning patterns, and make informed decisions about your treatment plan. Take the opportunity to discuss any questions or concerns you have regarding your readings to receive guidance and clarification.

By adhering to these guidelines for accuracy and consistency in blood pressure monitoring, you can rely on reliable and comparable readings. This empowers you to track your blood pressure effectively and facilitates productive discussions with your healthcare provider for optimal management of your cardiovascular health.

BLOOD PRESSURE LOGBOOK

Here is a sample logbook page designed for tracking your blood pressure measurements at home. This page offers designated spaces to record essential information, including the date, time, systolic and diastolic blood pressure readings, as well as heart rate.

By diligently completing this logbook page, you can effectively monitor your cardiovascular well-being, detect trends, and identify any recurring patterns. Remember to employ a trustworthy blood pressure monitor and adhere to correct measurement techniques.

Regularly sharing this logbook with your healthcare provider encourages fruitful discussions and enables informed decisions regarding your treatment plan. Embrace control over your health by utilizing this logbook to maintain a comprehensive overview of your blood pressure measurements.

Remember, by assuming command over your blood pressure through self-monitoring and making adjustments to your lifestyle, you have the power to substantially diminish the likelihood of complications and enhance your overall well-being. Through a suitable blend of medications, self-care practices, and consistent monitoring, you can effectively manage your blood pressure and enjoy an improved quality of life.

Time	Blood Pressure (mm Hg)		Heart Rate	Comments (e.g., activity change, diet change, medication change)
	Systolic (upper #)	Diastolic (lower #)		

CONCLUSION

Managing high blood pressure effectively can result in notable enhancements in health results. According to research by Yang et al. (2017), it was revealed that the utilization of medication and modifications in one's lifestyle, like shedding excess weight, engaging in physical activity, and employing stress management techniques, can lower the chances of developing heart disease, stroke, and other complications linked to elevated blood pressure The study also revealed that insufficient control of blood pressure was linked to weight gain, lack of physical activity, and excessive salt consumption.

This information emphasizes the significance of assuming responsibility for managing your blood pressure and collaborating closely with healthcare professionals to create a successful treatment strategy. By implementing a suitable combination of medications, lifestyle adjustments, and regular monitoring, individuals can substantially diminish their chances of experiencing complications and enjoy a healthier and more energetic life.

Don't wait for a health scare to take charge of your blood pressure. Start making small adjustments to your lifestyle today, such as incorporating exercise and adopting a heart-healthy diet. Work collaboratively with your healthcare providers to develop an effective treatment plan that suits your needs.

By doing so, you can significantly decrease the likelihood of heart disease, stroke, and other complications. Remember, taking control of your health is an ongoing journey. Stay proactive by monitoring your blood pressure regularly, staying updated on the latest research and treatment options, and seeking support from healthcare professionals and loved ones. Maintain your progress and embrace a healthy, happy life.

PAY IT FORWARD

WANT TO HELP OTHERS?

As we've said, knowledge is power... and this is your chance to spread it to help others.

Simply by sharing your honest opinion of this book and a little about your own experience, you'll show new readers that they're not alone and there's guidance out there to help them take control.

If you found this book valuable and insightful, I would greatly appreciate it if you could take a moment to leave a review. Thank you for your support and sharing your thoughts!

Scan to Leave a Review!

Follow Dr. Ashley Sullivan, PharmD on Facebook

And on her website **ashleysullivanonline.com**

REFERENCES

5 Steps to Quit Smoking. (2018). Www.heart.org. https://www.heart.org/en/healthy-living/healthy-lifestyle/quit-smoking-tobacco/5-steps-to-quit-smoking.

Alcohol and Heart Health: Separating Fact from Fiction. (n.d.). Www.hopkinsmedicine.org. https://www.hopkinsmedicine.org/health/wellness-and-prevention/alcohol-and-heart-health-separating-fact-from-fiction.

American Heart Association. (2017). Monitoring Your Blood Pressure at Home. Www.heart.org. https://www.heart.org/en/health-topics/high-blood-pressure/understanding-blood-pressure-readings/monitoring-your-blood-pressure-at-home.

Amin, M. (2020, January 9). Supplements vs Food: The Truth Behind Multi-Vitamins and Eating Right. Regenerate Medical Concierge. https://regeneratemedicalconcierge.com/supplements-vs-food-the-truth-behind-multi-vitamins-and-eating-right/.

Anderson, J. W., Liu, C., & Kryscio, R. J. (2008). Blood Pressure Response to Transcendental Meditation: A Meta-analysis. American Journal of Hypertension, 21(3), 310–316. https://doi.org/10.1038/ajh.2007.65.

Beckerman, J. (2021, September). The Link Between Drinking Alcohol and Heart Disease? WebMD. https://www.webmd.com/heart-disease/heart-disease-alcohol-your-heart

CDC. (2017, June 30). Benefits of Quitting. Centers for Disease Control and Prevention. https://www.cdc.gov/tobacco/quit_smoking/how_to_quit/benefits/index.htm.

BSc, K. G. (2023, May 17). Mediterranean Diet 101: A Meal Plan and Beginner's Guide. Healthline. https://www.healthline.com/nutrition/mediterranean-diet-meal-plan#menu-and-recipes.

Carol Dersarkissian. (2021). Slideshow: What Happens to Your Body

When You Quit Smoking.WebMD.https://www.webmd.com/smoking-cessation/ss/slideshow-effects-of-quitting-smoking.

CDC. (2020, November 9). 5 Surprising Facts About High Blood Pressure | cdc.gov. Centers for Disease Control and Prevention. https://www.cdc.gov/bloodpressure/5_surprising_facts.htm.

Cleveland Clinic. (2022, January 7). Blood Pressure: Treatments. Cleveland Clinic. https://my.clevelandclinic.org/health/diseases/17649-blood-pressure.

Contributors, W. E. (2023, April 29). Complementary vs. Alternative Medicine: What's the Difference? WebMD. https://www.webmd.com/balance/complementary-vs-alternative-medicine

Crouch, M. (2020, July 28). 7 Ways to Overcome Your Fitness Fears. AARP. https://www.aarp.org/health/healthy-living/info-2020/overcoming-fitness-fears.html.

D. Fryar, C., Ostchega, Y., M. Hales, C., Zhang, G., & Kruszon-Moran, D. (2019). Products - Data Briefs - Number 289 - October 2017. https://www.cdc.gov/nchs/products/databriefs/db289.htm.

DASH diet: Sample menus. (2023, May 31). Mayo Clinic. https://www.mayoclinic.org/healthy-lifestyle/nutrition-and-healthy-eating/in-depth/dash-diet/art-20047110.

Dekker, A. (2021, July 26). What are the effects of alcohol on the brain? Scientific American. https://www.scientificamerican.com/article/what-are-the-effects-of-a/

Eskarda. (2022, February 22). 6 Yoga Poses for High Blood Pressure. Yoga Journal. https://www.yogajournal.com/poses/yoga-by-benefit/high-blood-pressure/yoga-for-high-blood-pressure/.

Exercise: A drug-free approach to lowering high blood pressure. (2022, November 10). Mayo Clinic. https://www.mayoclinic.org/diseases-conditions/high-blood-pressure/in-depth/high-blood-pressure/art-20045206.

Francis, M. (2021, April 29). If slightly high blood pressure doesn't respond to lifestyle change, medication can help. American Heart Association. https://newsroom.heart.org/news/if-slightly-high-blood-pressure-doesnt-respond-to-lifestyle-change-medication-can-help.

Harvard Health. (2020, July 4). 11 ways to curb your drinking. Harvard Health. https://www.health.harvard.edu/staying-healthy/11-ways-to-curb-your-drinking.

Harvard Health Publishing. (2021). The benefits of do-it-yourself blood pressure monitoring. Harvard Health. https://www.health.harvard.edu/heart-health/the-benefits-of-do-it-yourself-blood-pressure-monitoring.

Harvard School of Public Health. (2016, April 12). Healthy Weight. The Nutrition Source. https://www.hsph.harvard.edu/nutrition source/healthy-weight/.

Hitti, M. (2013, August 22). 10 Relaxation Techniques That Zap Stress Fast. WebMD; WebMD. https://www.webmd.com/balance/guide/blissing-out-10-relaxation-techniques-reduce-stress-spot.

Houston, M. C., & Harper, K. J. (2008). Potassium, Magnesium, and Calcium: Their Role in Both the Cause and Treatment of Hypertension. The Journal of Clinical Hypertension, 10(7), 3–11. https://doi.org/10.1111/j.1751-7176.2008.08575.x.

Hypertension Prevalence in the U.S. | Million Hearts®. (2023, May 12). Centers for Disease Control and Prevention. https://million hearts.hhs.gov/data-reports/hypertension-prevalence.html.

L. Bhatt, D. (2022, May 1). Yoga and high blood pressure. Harvard Health. https://www.health.harvard.edu/heart-health/yoga-and-high-blood-pressure.

Landry, J. (2023, January 31). *72+ best hypertension quotes and sayings for inspiration (2023).* Respiratory Therapy Zone. https//www.respiratorytherapyzone.com/hypertension-quotes/

Landsbergis, P., Diez-Roux, A. V., Fujishiro, K., Baron, S., Kaufman, J. D., Meyer, J. S., Koutsouras, G. W., Shimbo, D., Shrager, S., Stukovsky, K. H., & Szklo, M. (2015). Job Strain, Occupational Category, Systolic Blood Pressure, and Hypertension Prevalence.

Journal of Occupational and Environmental Medicine, 57(11), 1178–1184. https://doi.org/10.1097/jom.0000000000000533.

Mawer, R. (2020, February 28). 17 Proven Tips to Sleep Better at Night. Healthline. https://www.healthline.com/nutrition/17-tips-to-sleep-better.

Mayo Clinic. (2015). Exercise: A drug-free approach to lowering high blood pressure. Mayo Clinic. https://www.mayoclinic.org/diseases-conditions/high-blood-pressure/in-depth/high-blood-pressure/art-20045206.

Mayo Clinic. (2021). How high blood pressure can affect your body. Mayo Clinic. https://www.mayoclinic.org/diseases-conditions/high-blood-pressure/in-depth/high-blood-pressure/art-20045868#

Miller, D. (2021). Complementary and Alternative Treatments for Hypertension. https://ruralhealth.und.edu/assets/4283-18665/treatments-for-hypertension.pdf

National Institute on Aging. (2021). Vascular Dementia: Causes, Symptoms, and Treatments. National Institute on Aging. https://www.nia.nih.gov/health/vascular-dementia.

NHS. (2019, February 11). Intensive blood pressure control may lessen cognitive loss. National Institutes of Health (NIH). https://www.nih.gov/news-events/nih-research-matters/intensive-blood-pressure-control-may-lessen-cognitive-loss#

Porter, E. (2017, November 14). Famous Faces of Heart Disease. Healthline. https://www.healthline.com/health/celebrities-with-heart-disease#david-letterman

Publishing, H. H. (2020, June 14). Meditation and a relaxation technique to lower blood pressure. Harvard Health. https://www.health.harvard.edu/heart-health/meditation-and-a-relaxation-technique-to-lower-blood-pressure.

Richter, A. (2020, December 23). 14 Supplements That May Help Lower Blood Pressure. Healthline. https://www.healthline.com/nutrition/supplements-lower-blood-pressure,

Salvetti, A., Brogi, G., Di Legge, V., & Bernini, G. P. (1993). The interrelationship between insulin resistance and hypertension. Drugs, 46 Suppl 2, 149–159. https://doi.org/10.2165/00003495-199300462-00024.

Schneider, J. K., Reangsing, C., & Willis, D. G. (2022). Effects of Transcendental Meditation on Blood Pressure. Journal of Cardiovascular Nursing, 37(3), E11–E21. https://doi.org/10.1097/jcn.0000000000000849.

Suni, E. (2021, March 10). How Much Sleep Do We Really Need? | National Sleep Foundation (A. Singh, Ed.). Sleep Foundation. https://www.sleepfoundation.org/how-sleep-works/how-much-sleep-do-we-really-need.

Tackling, G., & Borhade, M. B. (2022). Hypertensive Heart Disease. PubMed; StatPearls Publishing. https://www.ncbi.nlm.nih.gov/books/NBK539800/#:~:text=Hypertension%20disrupts%20the%20endothelial%20system.

U.S. Food and Drug Administration. (2022, June 2). FDA 101: Dietary Supplements. U.S. Food and Drug Administration. https://www.fda.gov/consumers/consumer-updates/fda-101-dietary-supplements.

W. Smith, M. (2021, September 20). Slideshow: 20 Foods That Can Save Your Heart. WebMD. https://www.webmd.com/heart-disease/ss/slideshow-foods-to-save-your-heart.

Wein, H. (2017, September 8). Understanding Health Risks. NIH News in Health. https://newsinhealth.nih.gov/2016/10/understanding-health-risks.

Why High Blood Pressure is a "Silent Killer." (2023, May 31). www.heart.org. https://www.heart.org/en/health-topics/high-blood-pressure/why-high-blood-pressure-is-a-silent-killer.

World Health Organization: WHO & World Health Organization: WHO. (2023). Hypertension. www.who.int. https://www.who.int/news-room/fact-sheets/detail/hypertension#

Yang, M. H., Kang, S. Y., Lee, J. A., Kim, Y. S., Sung, E. J., Lee, K.-Y.,

ROBORTROBORT

Kim, J.-S., Oh, H. J., Kang, H. C., & Lee, S. Y. (2017). The Effect of Lifestyle Changes on Blood Pressure Control among Hypertensive Patients. Korean Journal of Family Medicine, 38(4), 173. https://doi.org/10.4082/kjfm.2017.38.4.173.